The OMAD Diet

T0071957

The OMAD Diet

Intermittent Fasting WITH One Meal a Day TO Burn Fat AND Lose Weight

Alyssa Sybertz

ULYSSES PRESS

Text copyright © 2020 Alyssa Sybertz. Design and concept copyright © 2020 Ulysses Press and its licensors. All rights reserved. Any unauthorized duplication in whole or in part or dissemination of this edition by any means (including but not limited to photocopying, electronic devices, digital versions, and the internet) will be prosecuted to the fullest extent of the law.

Published in the United States by:
Ulysses Press
P.O. Box 3440
Berkeley, CA 94703
www.ulyssespress.com

ISBN: 978-1-64604-030-8
Library of Congress Catalog Number: 2020931883

Printed in the United States by Kingery Printing Company
10 9 8 7 6 5 4 3 2 1

Acquisitions editor: Casie Vogel
Managing editor: Claire Chun
Editor: Renee Rutledge
Proofreader: Kate St.Clair
Front cover design: David Hastings
Cover photo: © Davide Foti/Unsplash
Interior design: what!design @ whatweb.com

NOTE TO READERS: This book has been written and published strictly for informational and educational purposes only. It is not intended to serve as medical advice or to be any form of medical treatment. You should always consult your physician before altering or changing any aspect of your medical treatment and/or undertaking a diet regimen, including the guidelines as described in this book. Do not stop or change any prescription medications without the guidance and advice of your physician. Any use of the information in this book is made on the reader's good judgment after consulting with his or her physician and is the reader's sole responsibility. This book is not intended to diagnose or treat any medical condition and is not a substitute for a physician. This book is independently authored and published and no sponsorship or endorsement of this book by, and no affiliation with, any trademarked brands or other products mentioned within is claimed or suggested. All trademarks that appear in this book belong to their respective owners and are used here for informational purposes only. The author and publisher encourage readers to patronize the quality brands mentioned in this book.

For everyone who has been frustrated or discouraged in their attempts to lose weight: success is in your future, I know it!

Contents

Chapter 7
Giant Salads. 96

Chapter 8
One-Bowl Wonders 121

Chapter 9
Protein Plus Two 152

Chapter 10
Steaming Chilis and Soups 179

Chapter 11
Hearty Helpings 207

Introduction

The chorus of elated grunts grew louder. To watch the approaching throng, the women raised their heads above the bushes from which they were picking berries. The men were returning from the hunt, and it appeared they had been successful. A few of them dragged a large animal, perhaps a giant elk or even a woolly rhinoceros, nearer and nearer to where the women were gathered. Relief washed over them; finally, meat! After days, possibly weeks, of subsisting on tiny, tart fruits and tough root vegetables, they would eat their fill of energizing protein that night.

There has been plenty of debate over the types of foods our hunter-gatherer ancestors ate during the Paleolithic Period, and it is impossible to define one Paleolithic diet. The Hiwi people of Colombia and Venezuela ate primarily meat and fish, with 5% of their diet coming from fruits and vegetables, while the !Kung people of southern Africa enjoyed a diet made up of 60% nuts and seeds and only 10% meat and fish (both tribes continue to eat this way today).[1] But regardless of the differences in *what* they ate, there is a general agreement around *how* hunter-gatherers ate. Indeed, it is in their name: they survived by hunting, fishing, scavenging, and gathering. Due to their inability to produce food

---

1 Ferris Jabr, "How to Really Eat Like a Hunter-Gatherer: Why the Paleo Diet Is Half-Baked [Interactive & Infographic]," *Scientific American*, June 3, 2013, www.scientificamerican.com/article/why-paleo-diet-half-baked-how-hunter-gatherer-really-eat.

on their own, hunter-gatherers were entirely dependent on the abundance of game, fish, fruit, and/or plants in their region. If the weather changed abruptly and the plants perished or they were unable to make a kill, they would be forced to go without food. There was never any certainty around when or what the next meal would be. When food was plentiful, the Paleolithic people ate their fill. And when it was not, they fasted.

But even as agricultural practices evolved and grew, humans did not immediately begin eating three meals per day. The ancient Romans are believed to have enjoyed their largest (and sometimes only) meal in the afternoon or early evening, followed by a light supper before bed. Breakfast, for those who ate it, was often just a small bit of bread.[2] In ancient Japan, two meals a day was the norm, taken in late morning and early evening for the aristocrats and early morning and late evening for the laborers.[3] Later in history, in medieval England, the midday meal was the largest and often the only meal eaten in a day.[4]

Needless to say, the idea of eating three meals per day as a method of maintaining nourishment and fueling daily tasks did not evolve until thousands of years after the hunter-gatherers. In America particularly, the three-meal schedule only arose after the European settlers arrived. In fact, they held it up as an example of why they were more civilized than the Native Americans, who typically ate when they were hungry. Abigail Carroll, author of *Three Squares: The Invention of the American Meal*, has explained that the Europeans felt that putting boundaries and restrictions on

2 Mark Cartwright, "Food in the Roman World," *Ancient History Encyclopedia*, May 06, 2014, www.ancient.eu/article/684/food-in-the-roman-world.

3 Mark Cartwright, "Food & Agriculture in Ancient Japan," *Ancient History Encyclopedia*, June 20, 2017, www.ancient.eu/article/1082/food--agriculture-in-ancient-japan.

4 Mark Cartwright, "Leisure in an English Medieval Castle," *Ancient History Encyclopedia*, May 31, 2018, www.ancient.eu/article/1232/leisure-in-an-english-medieval-castle.

when they ate separated them from animals, who grazed and ate sporadically throughout the day.

The three-meal schedule arose out of necessity after the Industrial Revolution and the development of the nine-to-five workday. People began eating before they left for work, during their midday break, and after they returned home because the workday schedule dictated it, not because their stomachs were crying out to be fed on the appointed hour each day. Being part of a modern civilization ripe with industry meant establishing patterns and norms for the modern workday, and that included an eating pattern.

The growth of industry also gave way to one of the primary causes of the rise in obesity over the last century, particularly over the last sixty years. According to economists from Harvard University, increased production of processed and mass-prepared foods since the 1960s has led to people spending less time preparing meals, as well as an increase in the quantity and variety of food available, resulting in an increase in average caloric intake for many Americans.[5] Technological advances have also turned previously active jobs into more sedentary ones, simultaneously lowering caloric output. And obesity rates have risen accordingly, from 16% in 1971 to 30% in 1988 to 40% in 2016, according to the Centers for Disease Control and Prevention. At the same time, the risks of developing heart disease, high blood pressure, type 2 diabetes, osteoarthritis, and mental illness are rising. Yet Americans still continue to eat three meals per day.

Granted, many Americans eat and enjoy three meals every day and maintain a healthy weight. But nearly half of the population does not fall into this category, and cutting down from three meals a

---

5 David M. Cutler, et al., "Why Have Americans Become More Obese?" *Journal of Economic Perspectives* 17, no. 3 (2003): 93–118, doi:10.1257/089533003769204371.

day to just one might be the change they need to lose weight and improve their health. And that is where this book comes in.

Part 1 of this book details the science behind fasting and eating one meal a day, what exactly is going on in the body at the cellular level when food isn't being provided every few hours, and the research that has been done on the benefits of this system. You'll be provided with the tools and information you need to put together a single meal that fulfills all the daily nutritional requirements for a healthy, happy adult. Part 1 will also go into the healthy practices you can and should be doing during the fifteen waking hours in which you aren't enjoying your meal. This includes the foods and drinks that *are* allowed during your fasting period, as well as the best forms of exercise to complement eating just one meal a day. Throughout Part 1, you'll also see success stories based on interviews with real people who have tried the OMAD diet and how it has helped them meet their personal health and weight loss goals.

But before you start experimenting with your own meals, you can turn to Part 2 of this book, which is filled with over 100 delicious recipes specially designed to keep you healthy and energized when eaten as your only meal in a day. There are recipes for every taste and craving, from hearty one-bowl meals to huge, filling salads to sweet breakfast-style dishes. If you're keto, paleo, plant-based, or gluten-free, you will find recipes that fit within your dietary restrictions. Each recipe is accompanied by nutritional information to help you keep track of your daily macronutrient intake and ensure that eating one meal a day is not depriving you of any key nutrients nor stopping you from meeting your dietary needs.

I am not a trained chef, so the recipes in this book have been developed to be easy and approachable for the self-taught home cook. They don't require any fancy tools or equipment, or any ingredients you won't be able to find already in your cupboard or at your local grocery store. Cooking on an empty stomach might seem daunting, but these recipes are designed to take the stress out of that process.

This book is meant to serve as a guide, a jumping-off point for anyone interested in trying to eat just one meal a day. There are no required commitments, no set number of days you must follow the plan. There are no strict dietary restrictions in the recipes either. If you enjoy meat, you can choose meaty dishes. If you prefer a more plant-based diet, there are plenty of recipes for you as well. Eating just one meal a day can seem scary, intimidating, or impossible. As a health and nutrition writer, I have been offering people advice for years on the easiest and most effective ways to improve their health and well-being using diet and lifestyle changes. And I have come across countless different strategies, some certainly more compelling or promising than others. But as I researched this book, I became more and more convinced of the benefits of a fasting lifestyle. And I believe that when it is done intelligently and deliciously, it can be the key to unlocking a whole new level of health and happiness.

Part 1:
The Science of
the OMAD Diet

CHAPTER 1

The Science Behind Fasting

Physicians and healers throughout history have utilized fasting as a way to treat, heal, and cure various ailments. Hippocrates, the founder of modern medicine, commonly prescribed fasting as a treatment, as he believed it could "starve" disease. Research and medicine have come a long way since ancient Greece, but fasting has remained a tool in the physician's arsenal throughout the centuries. And today, researchers are uncovering exactly what is going on in the body during a fast and how that impacts the cellular and metabolic processes that make the body run.

When humans eat on a regular basis, cells rely on glucose, the simplest form of sugar, for energy. A meal is consumed, the food is broken down into its most basic components (for protein, this is amino acids; for fats, it's fatty acids; and for carbohydrates, it's glucose), and those components are transported through the bloodstream around the body—amino acids to the muscles to help maintain lean muscle mass, fatty acids to the brain, tissues, and organs to support healthy functioning, and glucose to cells all over to be utilized as fuel. Once the cells are essentially full, any remaining glucose from the meal is transported to the liver and muscles, where it is turned into glycogen, small bundles of glucose molecules, and stored.

If the cells run through their glucose and need more energy before the next meal, a signal goes out to the liver to break open the glycogen stores, turn them back into glucose, and send the glucose back out to the cells of the body. Regular, moderate consumption of carbohydrates will keep this cycle running constantly—glucose used, then stored, then used again. Weight gain commonly occurs when too many carbohydrates are consumed, because the body is getting a constant stream of new glucose to use for energy and never needs to break open the glycogen stores. In this case, the glycogen stores simply continue to grow, which translates to a bigger number on the scale.

While cells prefer to use glucose as fuel, they are capable of using fatty acids for the same purpose. However, the cells are programmed to use up any available glucose first before turning to fat, and this is where fasting comes in. A prolonged absence of carbohydrates forces the body to use up its glycogen stores. When the glycogen stores are depleted, the body is forced to turn to fat. In a fasted state, the body sends a signal to its fat cells to begin breaking down as an alternate fuel source. As they break down, they release both fatty acids and ketones, which are a by-product of the breakdown process. The fatty acids and ketones are then released into the body to provide fuel for the cells that have run out of glucose.

It does not take long for this switch to occur. A recent review led by Johns Hopkins University professor Mark Mattson and published in the journal *Ageing Research Reviews* looked at the changes in the levels of glucose and ketones in the body over the course of two days in response to three different eating patterns. High levels of glucose signal that the body is using it for fuel, while high levels of ketones denote that the body has made a switch and is using fat instead.

In subjects who followed a typical American eating pattern of three meals a day plus a late-evening snack (Group One), ketones remained consistently low while glucose spiked after every meal and remained relatively high throughout the day. In subjects who fasted for one whole day then ate three meals the next day (Group Two), glucose levels were low on the first day while ketones rose consistently until breakfast on the second day, when they dropped back down and glucose began to spike. Finally, Mattson looked at subjects who fasted for eighteen hours and restricted all their food consumption to a six-hour window in the afternoon (Group Three). In this case, glucose levels were elevated during and after the eating period, but ketones climbed during the last eight hours of the fasting period.[6]

Group Three is particularly noteworthy, especially as it pertains to only eating one meal a day. While ketone levels were elevated during the last eight hours of the fast in Group Two, they did not climb as high as they did in Group Three. So it stands to reason that if the fasting period were extended, ketone levels would continue to climb and glucose levels would remain low, meaning the body would break down even more fat to be used as fuel.

In addition to changing the body's primary fuel source, fasting can also alter the production of a few key hormones. Insulin is produced by the pancreas in response to carbohydrate consumption and facilitates the absorption and use of glucose by the cells. If there is consistently too much glucose in the bloodstream, due to overconsumption of carbohydrates, for example, the pancreas

---

6 Mark P. Mattson, et al., "Impact of Intermittent Fasting on Health and Disease Processes," *Ageing Research Reviews*, 39, (2017): 46–58, doi: 10.1016/j.arr.2016.10.005.

will flood the body with insulin to try to move the glucose out of the bloodstream and into the cells. Over time, the pancreas can get worn out and slow down insulin production, which can lead to problems like type 2 diabetes. But with fasting, the concentration of glucose in the bloodstream remains at a level that the pancreas can keep up with, keeping insulin production low and avoiding the development of conditions like type 2 diabetes and nonalcoholic fatty liver disease, in which fat accumulates in the liver and causes fatigue and inflammation.

Fasting can also directly affect the production of human growth hormone, or HGH. HGH plays a role in a number of bodily processes, including the growth of muscle and bone, the metabolism of sugar and fat, and the regulation of bodily fluids. However, HGH production in people who eat a standard three meals per day is inconsistent, which can lead to inefficiencies in these processes. Researchers from the University of Virginia School of Medicine found that fasting increases concentration of HGH by up to 210%, while researchers from the Intermountain Medical Center Heart Institute in Salt Lake City found that fasting for twenty-four hours can increase HGH levels by 1300% in women and 2000% in men, changes that can increase lean muscle mass, decrease fat mass, and maintain a steady metabolism.[7]

Once it became clear what exactly was happening in the body during a fast, researchers began to look at the specific impact fasting has on different conditions and areas of health research. The following sections describe some of the things they found.

---

7 K Y Ho, et al., "Fasting Enhances Growth Hormone Secretion and Amplifies the Complex Rhythms of Growth Hormone Secretion in Man," *The Journal of Clinical Investigation*, 81, no. 4 (1988): 968–975, doi:10.1172/JCI113450.

Weight Loss

A Czech study published in 2016 looked at the changes in body mass index (BMI), a common measure of body fat, in 48,673 individuals, specifically how those changes related to the number of meals each individual ate per day. They found that those who consumed only one meal a day saw the largest decrease in BMI, followed by those who ate two meals a day. In fact, the decrease in the one-meal-a-day (OMAD) group was double that of the two daily meals group, while the people who ate three or more meals per day actually saw an increase in BMI over the course of the study.[8]

Another study published in *The American Journal of Clinical Nutrition* aimed to see if shifting total daily food intake from three meals per day to one had any effect on various physical attributes, including body weight and body composition (or body fat mass). While the control group ate three daily meals designed for weight maintenance, the experimental group ate the same allotment of food, just confined to one meal, or one four-hour period in the early evening. Each group followed their appointed diet for eight weeks, followed by eleven weeks in which they ate whatever they wanted, and then they switched protocols. In the end, subjects experienced between a 2% and 10% decrease in weight and between a 13% and 24% decrease in body fat mass after eating just one meal a day. The group that ate three meals a day saw no change in body fat mass and a 1% increase in weight. When the study was published in 2007, the researchers speculated about the reason for these results, suspecting that the longer fast forced the body

---

8 Hana Kahleová, et al., "Frequency and Timing of Meals and Changes in Body Mass Index: Analysis of the Data from the Adventist Health Study-2," *Vnitrni Lekarstvi*, 62, no. 4 (2016): S15—20.

to break up fat deposits and use those fatty acids for energy, a suspicion that has since been confirmed in subsequent research.[9]

Type 2 Diabetes

A Canadian study published in the *World Journal of Diabetes* aimed to uncover the effects of intermittent fasting on subjects with type 2 diabetes. In it, the researchers encouraged the subjects to fast for up to eighteen to twenty hours daily for a period of two weeks and allowed them to eat anything they chose during the feeding period. The subjects, who were all taking medication for type 2 diabetes and on average were considered obese, self-reported their blood glucose levels, as well as their hours fasted, calories consumed, and any exercise. The findings showed significant group-wide decreases in weight, BMI, and morning glucose levels. Post-meal blood glucose levels also improved during the fasting period by 8%. Furthermore, 34% of participants hit their target fasting blood sugar levels, while only 13% hit them prior to the study. Sixty percent of the participants said they would continue with the intermittent fasting regimen after the study was over. "A strong association between the increase in hours fasted from baseline, and the probability of attaining a normal fasting glucose level was found," wrote the researchers, suggesting that if participants were able to prolong the fast beyond the average reported fast of twelve hours per day, the benefits would be even more pronounced.[10]

American researchers published in the journal *Cell Metabolism* took a slightly different approach, studying how intermittent fasting

---

9 Kim S. Stone, et al., "A Controlled Trial of Reduced Meal Frequency without Caloric Restriction in Healthy, Normal-Weight, Middle-Aged Adults," *American Journal of Clinical Nutrition*, 85, no.4 (2007): 981—988, doi:10.1093/ajcn/85.4.981.

10 Terra G. Arnason, et al., "Effects of Intermittent Fasting on Health Markers in Those with Type 2 Diabetes: A Pilot Study," *World Journal of Diabetes*, 8, no. 4: 15464—164, doi:10.4239/wjd. v8.i4.154.

impacted key markers of the onset of type 2 diabetes, such as insulin sensitivity and β cell responsiveness (how efficiently the cells of the pancreas are producing insulin), in subjects with pre-diabetes. Participants' eating was confined to a six-hour period in the morning, and the food provided was meant to promote weight maintenance, not loss. The study found that this fasting protocol decreased fasting and post-meal insulin levels, as well as average and peak insulin levels by 1200% and 33% respectively, plus improved β cell responsiveness and decreased insulin resistance (when cells don't respond to insulin, preventing glucose from being absorbed and utilized) by 350%. The researchers also noted that these improvements did not disappear immediately after the subjects went back to their normal eating patterns and meal choices, suggesting that a period of intermittent fasting may have long-lasting benefits even after being discontinued.[11]

OMAD SUCCESS STORY: KIMBERLY, 35

Kimberly had been overweight since she was six years old. At twenty-five, she weighed 370 pounds, had sleep apnea, and couldn't stand or walk without pain. She lost her job because she couldn't bear to venture out of the house, and at one point caught herself feeling at peace with dying before she reached thirty, which scared and frustrated her. She had tried multiple weight-loss strategies in the past, like cutting calories, eating frozen diet meals such as Lean Cuisine, and only eating oatmeal. They would work for a time and she would lose a little weight, but she was constantly starving and could never sustain the lifestyle. There were numerous moments over the years in which Kimberly knew she needed to find

11 Elizabeth F. Sutton, et al., "Early Time-Restricted Feeding Improves Insulin Sensitivity, Blood Pressure, and Oxidative Stress Even without Weight Loss in Men with Prediabetes," *Cell Metabolism*, 27, no. 6 (2018): 1212–1221, doi:10.1016/j.cmet.2018.04.010.

the strategy that would work for her, but she didn't know what it was or how to find it.

One morning, Kimberly woke up particularly hungry and decided to eat all of her calories for the day at breakfast. Hunger was always Kimberly's biggest struggle when trying to stick to a diet plan, but to her surprise, she wasn't hungry when dinnertime rolled around that day. She quickly found that enjoying one big meal was much easier for her than eating three small ones throughout the day. She hopped online to see if this way of eating was healthy and discovered that it was not only healthy, but it was also a way of eating called OMAD that people had been doing for thousands of years.

So Kimberly stuck with eating one meal a day. In the morning she would eat eggs, oatmeal, vegetables, or veggie powder mixed with water. Throughout the day she would drink water and black coffee, taking care to keep her food intake below 50 calories so as not to break the fast. Today, Kimberly has lost 150 pounds, a journey she has chronicled on Instagram and YouTube @kimberfitgirl. Her skin and hair look younger and more radiant, and she no longer struggles with hunger. Even better, OMAD works great with Kimberly's busy work schedule, making her day-to-day life easier. OMAD is the only thing that ever brought Kimberly real, sustainable weight-loss results, and she now has every intention of living a long, healthy, happy life.

Heart Health

A study published in the journal *Annals of Nutrition and Metabolism* looked at the effects of fasting—specifically, the twelve-hour Ramadan fast—on a number of key risk factors of cardiovascular disease. These included homocysteine (an amino acid found mostly in meat that has been linked to heart disease), interleukin-6 (an inflammatory molecule produced by the immune system), C-reactive protein (a protein whose concentration in the body increases in response to an increase in inflammation), and the ratio of total cholesterol to HDL (good) cholesterol, a number that can predict atherosclerosis, the buildup of plaque in the arteries that can restrict blood flow to the heart. The researchers tested the levels of all of these markers prior to the fast, after four weeks of fasting, and three weeks after the fast was complete. They found that levels of homocysteine, interleukin-6, and C-reactive protein all decreased after fasting by up to 26%, 60%, and 50%, respectively. The total cholesterol to HDL ratio also decreased at the end of the fast and three weeks after, from 3.56 to 2.47 in males and from 3.45 to 2.12 in females. The optimal ratio is 3.5 or below, with anything over 5.0 signaling a greater chance of developing heart disease.[12]

Brain Health

Research from Saudi Arabia published in 2018 looked at the effects of fasting until the evening on levels of a neurotransmitter called orexin-A, which plays a key role in regulating feelings of wakefulness and can affect focus and sleep cycles. They found that levels of orexin-A were lower at night and higher in the daytime during fasting, with daytime levels nearly double that of the control group, which ate three regular daily meals. This suggests that contrary to some beliefs, fasting does not increase feelings of sleepiness or grogginess during the day.[13]

---

12 Fehime B. Aksungar, et al., "Interleukin-6, C-Reactive Protein, and Biochemical Parameters during Prolonged Intermittent Fasting," *Annals of Nutrition & Metabolism*, 51, no. 1 (2007): 88—95, doi: 10.1159/000100954.

13 Aljohara S. Almeneessier, et al., "The Effects of Diurnal Intermittent Fasting on the Wake-Promoting Neurotransmitter Orexin-A," *Annals of Thoracic Medicine*, 13, no. 1 (2018): 48—54, www.ncbi.nlm.nih.gov/pmc/articles/PMC5772108.

While research in humans is limited, there have been a number of studies in mice linking fasting diets to improvements in memory, cognitive function, and Alzheimer's disease. One study published in the journal *PLOS One* found that mice subjected to an alternate-day fasting diet saw improvements in learning and memory compared to mice who were fed a high-fat diet.[14] A Chinese study from 2017 looked specifically at the proteins in the brain that cause Alzheimer's disease, both in the brains of mice and in vitro. It found that alternate-day fasting altered the concentrations of these proteins and how they interact with one another in a way that exhibited beneficial effects against Alzheimer's. The researchers explained that most of the medications available today work to slow or stop the progression of Alzheimer's, but intermittent fasting could be a way to prevent it.[15]

Cancer

Doctors at UC San Diego's Moores Cancer Center published a study in 2016 aiming to determine whether the duration of the nightly fast impacts the likelihood of breast cancer recurrence in women. After analyzing data reported by 2,413 women over a four-year period and following up with them an average of seven to eleven years later, they discovered that fasting for fewer than thirteen hours per night was associated with a 36% higher risk of breast cancer recurrence compared to fasting for more than thirteen hours per night. They also found that each two-hour increase in the duration of the fast was associated with a lower level of

14 Liaoliao Li, et al., "Chronic Intermittent Fasting Improves Cognitive Functions and Brain Structures in Mice," *The Public Library of Science 8, no.6 (2013), doi: 10.1371/journal. pone.00660069.*

15 Jingzhu Zhang, et al., "Intermittent Fasting Protects Against Alzheimer's Disease Possible through Restoring Aquaporin-4 Polarity," *Frontiers in Molecular Neuroscience* 10, no. 395 (2019), doi:10.3389/fnmol.2017.00395.

hemoglobin A1c, a marker of diabetes risk that has been linked to increased likelihood of developing cancer.[16]

In addition to helping prevent the development of cancer, fasting can help those going through treatment as well. According to a review in the journal *Cell Cycle,* scientists from the University of Southern California looked at the severity of the side effects of chemotherapy in cancer patients who fasted before treatment compared to patients who did not. They found reductions in symptom severity across the board, with the most notable being the total disappearance of vomiting and diarrhea, an 80% decrease in nausea, a 67% decrease in dry mouth, a 56% decrease in fatigue, and a 53% decrease in feelings of weakness.[17]

* * *

Data continues to pour in on the effects of different forms of fasting, but it is becoming increasingly clear that even occasional brief fasts can have major benefits on multiple levels of health. And the reason boils down to this: When humans are constantly eating, the body is constantly forced to react and respond to the food that is being consumed, and to figure out how best to utilize it. But when eating is interrupted, the body can take time to evaluate the resources it has and determine how best to utilize them in order to move itself toward a state of optimal health.

To be sure, food is a necessity for survival. Nutrients are essential for maintaining the production of the hormones and chemicals that keep all bodily processes running. Without food, these processes will eventually slow and break down. And fasting is not ideal for people with certain health conditions, such as low blood sugar or

16 Catherine R. Marinac, et al., "Prolonged Nightly Fasting and Breast Cancer Prognosis," *JAMA Oncology,* 2, no.8 (2016): 1049—55, doi:10.1001/jamanoncol.2016.0164.

17 Lizzia Raffaghello, et al., "Fasting and Differential Chemotherapy Protection in Patients," *Cell Cycle* 15, no.22 (2010): 4474—6, doi:10.4161/cc.9.22.13954.

diabetes, or those who are taking certain medications, such as those for blood pressure or heart disease. It is important to discuss it with your doctor or health care practitioner if you are considering trying fasting. But if your health permits, daily fasts, especially those longer than twelve hours, are continually proving to provide the body with all the fuel it needs while also giving it time to achieve a state of homeostasis that will optimize health.

CHAPTER 2

Building Your One Meal a Day

Some proponents of the OMAD diet say that everything you need to know about the diet is in the name: you eat one meal a day. That's it. It does not matter what's on your plate, as long as you are only sitting down to eat once every twenty-four hours. And, to be sure, this approach has its supporters. There are people who love OMAD for this very reason, because they don't need to count calories or measure out portion sizes or go out of their way to purchase healthy ingredients. Only eating once a day gives them the freedom to eat whatever they want.

This approach will yield some results, as the body will still enter a state during the fast in which it is burning fat for fuel instead of glucose, but the risks can outweigh these benefits. Eating anything and everything during the one meal, which some folks take as a free pass to enjoy not-so-healthy foods, can yield deficiencies in macro and micronutrients that are critical to maintaining the body's life-sustaining processes. Increased feelings of hunger also make it likely that you'll consume even more of these unhealthy foods than you would have if you were eating more than one meal a day.

That said, if you've picked up this book, chances are you want to take a different approach to OMAD, one in which the fast is sustainable and enjoyable at the same time. The primary concern for most newcomers to this way of eating is hunger. As in, how will it not consume your mind and body for every moment in which you aren't eating. The keys to warding off hunger during the twenty-three hours of not eating lie in the practices surrounding the one meal. More specifically, what is on the plate and how it is eaten.

Food serves one primary purpose: to provide fuel for the cells of the body. Within food, there are three primary macronutrients: fats, carbohydrates, and protein. Each provides a unique type of fuel. The ways that fats and carbohydrates serve as fuel were discussed in Chapter 1 (beginning on page 8). The third macronutrient, protein, is capable of serving as a fuel source in the same way as its macronutrient counterparts, but its primary role is to serve as a building block for tissues and muscles. Essentially, all tissues and muscles can be broken down into tiny amino acids, the most basic components of protein. In order to keep the cells running efficiently during the fast, when food is not being consumed, a sufficient amount of each of these macronutrients must be provided in the day's only meal. These benchmark amounts, which are based off of the Food and Drug Administration's recommended dietary allowance of each, can help you construct a meal that will keep you full and energized throughout the day.

The recipes in Part 2 of this book were developed with these benchmarks in mind, and as such are a superb place to start when beginning OMAD. Each one is accompanied by nutritional information that reveals how much of each macronutrient is present in the meal. What follows here is a breakdown of each macronutrient, the role it plays in sustaining an OMAD diet, and the foods that provide it in the highest amounts.

Protein

Countless studies have looked at what makes a food filling and which foods increase and extend feelings of satiety the most. A 2016 review published in the *Journal of the Academy of Nutrition and Dietetics* found that eating high-protein foods after a fast increases feelings of fullness over a longer period of time than other foods.[18] Indeed, the popularity of diets like Atkins in the early 2000s and paleo in the 2010s proves that when people want to eat less, they increase their protein intake. One of the primary reasons for this is protein's effect on levels of the hormone ghrelin. Known as the "hunger hormone," ghrelin signals to the brain that it is time to eat, which then causes feelings of hunger. In the past, ghrelin's purpose was strictly one of survival, while today it is one of the primary reasons that people fail to lose weight when they diet. But researchers from Israel found that a high-protein meal reduced ghrelin levels by 45%, plus significantly reduced feelings of hunger and cravings. These effects also led to continuous weight loss for the study subjects over the course of thirty-two weeks, while the group that wasn't eating high-protein meals experienced an eventual regain.[19]

The FDA's daily recommended protein intake is 50 grams. The majority of the recipes in this book have at least 50 grams of protein per serving, and many of them have more. A few of the meat-free recipes, like the Frittata Primavera (page 82) and the Garlicky Pasta with Eggplant, Artichokes, and Mushrooms (page 226) have fewer than 50 grams of protein but feature indulgent ingredients like cheeses and large portion sizes that help boost

---

18 Jaapna Dhillon, et al., "The Effects of Increased Protein Intake on Fullness: A Meta-Analysis and Its Limitations," *Journal of the Academy of Nutrition and Dietetics* 116, no. 6 (2016): 968–983. doi: 10.1016/j.jand.2016.01.003.

19 Daniela Jakubowicz, et al., "Meal Timing and Composition Influence Ghrelin Levels, Appetite Scores and Weight Loss Maintenance in Overweight and Obese Adults," *Steroids* 77, no. 4 (2012): 323–331. doi:10.1016/j.steroids.2011.12.006.

satiety. That said, one or more protein-rich ingredients is vital to include in an OMAD meal. Here are some of the best ones:

- Beef (52 grams per 6 ounces)
- Chicken (49 grams per 6 ounces)
- Turkey (47 grams per 6 ounces)
- Salmon (44 grams per 6 ounces)
- Protein powder (44 grams per 2 scoops)
- Pork (38 grams per 6 ounces)
- Quinoa (12 grams per ½ cup)
- Greek yogurt (10 grams per ½ cup)
- Peanuts (9 grams per ¼ cup)
- Peanut butter (8 grams per 2 tablespoons)
- Black beans (8 grams per ½ cup)
- Walnuts (8 grams per ¼ cup)
- Kidney beans (7 grams per ½ cup)
- Chickpeas (6 grams per ½ cup)
- Eggs (6 grams per egg)
- Almonds (5 grams per ¼ cup)

OMAD SUCCESS STORY: WENDY, 68

For the better part of her adult life, Wendy was a type 2 diabetic and a yo-yo dieter. After fighting and beating cancer in her late fifties, Wendy's weight peaked at 180 pounds on her 5'3" frame, and she began to give up emotionally. Her father and her sister had both passed away from complications from diabetes, her father at 51 and her sister at 70, and both had been on insulin. So when her doctor told her she too needed insulin to control her fasting glucose levels, which had reached 300 when they should have been under 100, it was a wake-up call for Wendy. She didn't want to go down that same path.

Wendy started doing research online and came across some information on the keto diet. Her body had never reacted well to carbs, so the eating plan seemed promising. She started eating more fats and fewer carbs. The scale began to trend downward, but after two months of keto, Wendy never felt quite right. She knew that there had to be something else she could do to take her health to the next level.

That was when she realized that mealtimes would arrive and she wouldn't be hungry. In her research Wendy had found some information on OMAD, and now she wondered if that was the ticket. She started gradually stretching out the time between her meals, fasting for eighteen hours a day and enjoying two meals in the remaining six. But even then, she never felt hungry, so she stretched her fast to twenty hours and then to 23.

Wendy began eating one meal around 1:00 p.m. daily. Her meal would be a 14-ounce ribeye steak cooked in butter, or salmon, or eggs. Sometimes she would make a big roast and then portion it out to eat for a few days. She would enjoy a butter coffee in the morning, blending grass-fed butter, coconut oil, and sometimes a teaspoon of unsweetened cocoa powder into her coffee, then drink water or black tea throughout the day.

Wendy lost 40 pounds in the first four months and 50 pounds after six months. Her fasting glucose level plummeted from 300 to 80, and she was able to stop taking insulin. Her complexion is brighter, she's sleeping better, and her energy levels are higher than they've been in twenty years. Wendy realized that she had been forcing herself to eat three meals a day, and now that she's only eating one, she feels lighter, healthier, and happier than ever before.

Carbohydrates

When it comes to changing an eating plan or going on a diet, carbs are almost always the most hotly contested subject for two key reasons. One is that reducing carbohydrate intake will help the majority of people lose weight. And two is that for the majority of people, carbs are the most difficult to give up. Bread, pastries, cookies, pasta, and pancakes are mood-boosting comfort foods, and giving them up causes some people so much distress that even if they do see results on the scale, emotionally it isn't worth it. Eating just once a day can already be difficult mentally, and for that reason, the recipes in this book are not all low carb. Many of them, such as the salads and egg recipes, are naturally low carb, while others use certain types of pastas and breads. And that is because there is another nutrient that is technically a carbohydrate that can be tremendously beneficial on OMAD. That nutrient is fiber.

Fiber

Apart from protein, fiber plays the largest role in promoting feelings of satiety after a meal. Fiber is not digested by the human body, but it does slow down the movement of food through the digestive tract, prolonging feelings of fullness as it does so. There are two types of fiber: soluble and insoluble. Soluble fiber dissolves in water, creating a gel-like substance in the colon that slows the digestion and absorption of the other foods being digested. Insoluble fiber is not broken down at all and moves through the GI tract intact, creating a feeling of the stomach being physically full. Most of the foods that contain fiber, such as vegetables, legumes, and whole grains, contain a combination of both types.

In addition to increasing feelings of fullness, fiber, particularly soluble fiber, has other effects that promote weight loss. As it slows the absorption of nutrients from foods into the bloodstream, soluble fiber keeps fat from being absorbed and stored and sugars from being absorbed and spiking blood sugar levels. It is also the preferred food source for the beneficial bacteria living in the gut, meaning that a high-fiber diet can help maintain the balanced microbiome that plays a critical role in virtually all health-promoting processes. Researchers from the University of Kentucky's medical school found that increased fiber intake can lower blood pressure, improve cholesterol levels, improve insulin sensitivity, boost immunity, and lower instances of many gastrointestinal disorders.[20] Meanwhile, a 2019 meta-analysis commissioned by the World Health Organization discovered that people who ate the most fiber were up to 30% less likely to die prematurely from any cause, while a fiber-rich diet was correlated with up to a 24% lower incidence of heart disease, stroke, type 2 diabetes, and colon cancer.[21]

The FDA's recommendation for daily fiber intake is 25 grams. Many of the recipes in this book contain at least that much fiber, if not more. Others, like the Chocolate Almond Loaded Oatmeal (page 86) and the Chicken Marsala with Nutty Veggie Bowties (page 216), contain around 15 grams of fiber. The reason: High-fiber ingredients do not lend themselves to every cuisine, and the meals in this book are meant to be delicious as well as nutritious. But on days when you're craving one of the recipes that contain slightly less fiber, there are easy ways to increase your total intake (more details on those later in the chapter). Here are some of the foods you will see in the recipes that deliver the most fiber:

---

20 J. W. Anderson, et al., "Health Benefits of Dietary Fiber," *Nutrition Reviews* 67, no. 4 (2009): 188–205.

21 Andrew Reynolds, et al., "Carbohydrate Quality and Human Health: A Series of Systematic Reviews and Meta-Analyses," *The Lancet* 393, no. 10160 (2019): 434–445.

- Whole wheat pasta (15 grams per 6 ounces)
- Black beans (8 grams per ½ cup)
- Flax seeds (7 grams per tablespoon)
- Kidney beans (7 grams per ½ cup)
- Avocado (7 grams per half)
- Quinoa (6 grams per ½ cup)
- Chia seeds (5 grams per tablespoon)
- Chickpeas (5 grams per ½ cup)
- Oats (4 grams per ½ cup)
- White and sweet potatoes (4 grams per potato)
- Almonds (3 grams per ¼ cup)
- Brown rice (3 grams per ½ cup)
- Walnuts (2 grams per ¼ cup)

Fruits and Vegetables

Fruits and vegetables are an essential part of any diet and can be a boon to anyone on OMAD. In addition to providing a plethora of beneficial vitamins, minerals, and other plant compounds (like antioxidants, compounds that protect and strengthen cells) that can't be obtained through the other foods mentioned thus far, plants can be used to add satiating bulk to meals. Crunchy veggies require more work and more time to chew, prolonging eating time and increasing feelings of fullness. Fruits and veggies also work in a variety of ways to tamp down inflammation, a condition that is widely considered to be one of the primary causes behind everything from weight gain to heart disease.

The larger variety of colors you choose in your fruits and vegetables, the larger variety of powerful antioxidants you will consume.

Bright red tomatoes and bell peppers deliver lycopene, which helps protect the heart. Orange and yellow carrots, peppers, and mangoes contain beta-carotene, a compound the body converts to vitamin A to keep the eyes healthy and strengthen the immune system. Broccoli, leafy greens, asparagus, Brussels sprouts and green beans owe their green color to chlorophyll, the compound that helps plants convert sunlight to energy and provides many benefits for humans, including supporting the body's detoxification, energy, and immune processes. The bluish/purple hues of blueberries, blackberries, red grapes, beets, and red onions mean that these foods contain anthocyanins, antioxidants that help prevent the spread of dangerous fat around the organs.

The recipes in this book are filled with whole fruits and vegetables. Many are fresh, while some are frozen. When purchasing frozen fruits and vegetables, be sure that nothing has been added to them before freezing. If they were frozen immediately after being picked, they will deliver the same amount of beneficial nutrients as their fresh counterparts.

A Note on Sugar

When people talk about the negative impact that carbs have on your diet, they are more than likely talking about sugar. Indeed, many foods that are high in carbohydrates, such as bread and other baked goods, are made up mostly of sugar (or glucose). When sugar is consumed, the body will immediately try to use it as a source of fuel—but in most instances, there is too much of it to be used immediately, so it is stored. If this process is repeated without the stores ever being utilized, as was discussed in Chapter 1, more and more sugar will continue to be stored, resulting in more and more weight gain. In addition, continuous sugar consumption causes constant rises and falls in blood sugar levels, resulting in changes in mood, cravings, and energy levels. Blood sugar fluctuations are a main cause of overeating and the eventual development of insulin resistance and type 2 diabetes.

But for people who want to eat a well-rounded, well-balanced diet, it is hard to escape sugar all together. Many fruits are high in sugar, so much so that proponents of some eating plans advocate eliminating fruit altogether. And while this would drastically reduce sugar intake, it would also drastically reduce intake of the many healthy vitamins, minerals, and antioxidants that fruits deliver. One of the best ways to tackle this quandary is to differentiate between added sugar, or sugar that has been added to processed foods, and natural sugars, or those that exist in whole foods. As a rule, try to avoid processed foods that contain added sugar, but enjoy fruits. The best way to do so when only eating one meal a day is to make sure the meal also contains ingredients that are high in fiber, like in the Tropical Smoothie Bowl (page 84). That way, the sugars that are present are absorbed slowly and you can avoid the craving-inducing blood sugar spikes that can make OMAD more difficult.

Fats

Just as there are healthy carbohydrates (fiber-rich foods and antioxidant-rich fruits) and unhealthy carbohydrates (sugar-packed cookies and pastries) there are healthy and unhealthy fats, and it is important to consider the differences when deciding which fats to include in your meal. This is true even if you are eating a high-fat, low-carb diet, as certain types of fats are not going to fuel your body in the same way as others. The group of fats that doctors and scientists agree should be avoided is artificial trans fats, which are created when vegetable oil is altered to stay solid at room temperature, a technique that gives processed and commercially produced foods a longer shelf life. Artificial trans fats have been shown to increase levels of LDL (bad) cholesterol, increase inflammation and the diseases it causes, and boost chances of developing insulin resistance and type 2 diabetes.

Advice tends to be mixed when it comes to saturated fats, the type of fat found in red meat, whole milk dairy, cheese, coconut oil, and many processed foods. Saturated fats have been linked to increases in total cholesterol, but recent meta-analyses have concluded that there is not enough evidence to directly link high saturated fat intake with increased risk for conditions like heart disease. Instead, experts suggest replacing at least some of the saturated fats in your diet with unsaturated fats, the type found mostly in plant-based foods and oils.

Two types of unsaturated fat, monounsaturated and polyunsaturated, are considered healthy fats. These are the fats that the body needs to perform essential processes and that have been linked to lower blood pressure and increased levels of HDL (good) cholesterol. One type of polyunsaturated fat in particular, omega-3, has been linked to numerous health benefits. A study in the journal *Brain, Behavior, and Immunity* linked a higher intake of omega-3s to lower levels of inflammation and anxiety, while researchers from Greece found that omega-3s can help heal a fatty liver.[22, 23] Scientists at Massachusetts General Hospital and Harvard Medical School even found that subjects who consumed omega-3 fatty acids had a lower risk for a cardiac event, stroke, or cardiac death.[24]

---

22 Janice Kiecolt-Glaser, et al., "Omega-3 Supplementation Lowers Inflammation and Anxiety in Medical students; A Randomized Controlled Trial," *Brain, Behavior, and Immunity* 25, no. 8 (2011): 1725–1734. doi:10.1016/j.bbi.2011.07.229.

23 Dimitrios Bouzianas, et al., "Potential Treatment of Human Nonalcoholic Fatty Liver Disease with Long-Chain Omega-3 Polyunsaturated Fatty Acids," *Nutrition Reviews* 71, no. 11 (2013): 753–771. doi:10.1111/nure.12073.

24 Alexander Leaf, "Historical Overview of n-3 Fatty Acids and Coronary Heart Disease," *American Journal of Clinical Nutrition* 87, no. 6 (2008): 1978S–1980S.

The FDA's daily recommended dietary allowance for fat is 65 grams. The fat content of the recipes in this book varies pretty widely depending on the ingredients. Salads that are dressed with an olive oil–based dressing, like the Salmon and Strawberry Salad (page 102), tend to have more fat than recipes like the Apple Cinnamon Loaded Oatmeal (page 87) or the Hummus and Falafel Bowl (page 128). But, in general, these are the ingredients that can be utilized to add health-promoting unsaturated fats:

- Avocado (20 grams per half)
- Walnuts (18 grams per ¼ cup)
- Peanuts (18 grams per ¼ cup)
- Peanut butter (16 grams per 2 tablespoons)
- Olive oil (14 grams per tablespoon)
- Salmon (14 grams per 8 ounces)
- Coconut oil (12 grams per tablespoon)
- Almonds (12 grams per ¼ cup)
- Flax seeds (9 grams per tablespoon)
- Chia seeds (4 grams per tablespoon)
- Eggs (4 grams per egg)

OMAD SUCCESS STORY: KAY, 35

Growing up, Kay was always athletic and thin and didn't worry much about her weight. So when she became pregnant with her daughter in 2012, she assumed she would just put on weight during her pregnancy and then it would come off. But when her daughter turned two and Kay was still carrying around her extra pregnancy weight, she decided it was time to do something about it.

The only problem: Nothing worked. Kay tried Weight Watchers, juice cleanses, caloric restriction, frozen diet meals, and exercising multiple times a day. She was putting in 100% effort, but nothing was changing. In fact, there were times when Kay would lose 2 pounds and then quickly gain 8 for reasons she couldn't see. Eventually, her weight peaked at 189 pounds. She was flummoxed and frustrated.

In 2016, Kay felt like she'd had enough. The only thing she hadn't tried, the thing she had considered a last resort, was to simply not eat. Kay loved to eat and especially loved to snack so she was skeptical that fasting would be sustainable. Even so, she started doing research and seeing the results that others were experiencing, which convinced her that she had to give it a shot. All she needed to do was change when she ate, not what she ate.

Kay decided to start with 16:8 intermittent fasting. She would stop eating at 8:00 p.m. and wait to eat again until 12:00 p.m. the following day. She cut out cake and soda, but otherwise continued to eat the foods she enjoyed, which often consisted of a huge, fresh salad for lunch. She never felt guilty about portion sizes or even what she was eating, sometimes heading to Chick-Fil-A if that was what she was craving. Kay didn't actively decide to extend her fast, but her hunger at dinnertime slowly began to disappear. She went from having a meal to snacking on some popcorn to skipping eating altogether. Feeling empowered, she extended her fast to 20 hours, delighted by how it took the stress out of finding time to eat multiple meals on busy days.

Kay lost 33 pounds over her first year of fasting, dropping to 156 pounds. She enjoys exercising and was worried she wouldn't have the energy, but actually improved her fitness over that time. She is less dependent on coffee to get her through the day and is much more in control of her cravings for sweets. Kay used to suffer from asthma and Crohn's disease but has not had a flare-up or an incident since she began fasting. She also found herself saving money because she wasn't purchasing snacks throughout the day. Today, Kay continues to fast and share her journey at GoodGirlGoneOMAD.com. After countless failures, Kay believes she has finally found the eating plan that will be healthy, easy, and sustainable for her going forward.

When to Eat

Just as societal and lifestyle changes led to the rise in the three-meals-a-day eating model, your lifestyle, schedule, and personal eating preferences can dictate the time of day you choose to enjoy your one meal a day. For folks who feel starved after waking up, the meal can be eaten in the morning to offer sustained energy throughout the day. For those whose hunger starts to peak around midday or who have a job that sends them out of the house for the evening and overnight hours, eating the meal around lunchtime might be the best choice. And for those who prefer to fast throughout the morning and afternoon with the prospect of a hearty meal coming in the evening, dinnertime may be ideal. Choice of mealtime can also depend on when you have the most time to sit down and enjoy your one meal (more on this in the next section).

Success with OMAD does not rely on when you eat your one meal a day. In fact, it is one of the things that makes the diet so simple. Most of the benefits for weight loss come during the 23-hour fast, not the 1 hour in which you are eating. As long as the fast lasts for 23 hours, it does not matter which 23 hours in the 24-hour cycle those are. However, to get the maximum benefits, mealtime should be consistent each day to ensure that the fast is in fact 23 hours long. If you're just starting out with OMAD and unsure of what time of day to eat, feel free to experiment a bit with different mealtimes at first. But the faster you can find a schedule that works for you and stick to it, the faster you will see results.

Eating Mindfully

When eating only one meal a day, it can be tempting to inhale said meal the second it touches your plate. However, doing so will only make sticking to the plan more difficult. Thousands of Americans eat on the go, in their cars or as they're walking out the door. If you're only eating once a day, you deserve to set aside enough time in your busy schedule to sit down and actually eat that meal. How you eat your meal during this time will help you find that much more success with OMAD.

If you've read anything about health and wellness in the last few years, you've likely heard about a practice called mindfulness. Mindfulness is the idea of being present, of taking the time to notice everything, from your surroundings to your breathing. The most common mindfulness practice is mindfulness meditation, which has exploded in popularity because of how it helps people overcome stress, be more productive, and improve mental health overall. The practice of mindful eating applies this approach to mealtime, suggesting that you utilize all of the senses to enjoy a meal—seeing the colors and shapes of the food on your plate, smelling the aromas, hearing the crunch or the sizzle, feeling the heft of a bite on your fork and, finally, tasting the flavors. It involves chewing each bite slowly and feeling the way the food breaks down in your mouth. It is about recognizing and listening to your body's responses to the food. When you're eating mindfully, you are only eating, not trying to multitask or read or watch TV. And applying these practices to cooking as well as to eating can make the entire process of preparing and savoring your one meal that much more satisfying. OMAD is not about depriving yourself of enjoying a meal. Instead, it can be an opportunity to enjoy it even more.

Many studies have been conducted to examine the benefits of mindful eating as it relates to weight loss, cravings, and disordered eating. A Dutch study published in the journal *Appetite* found that individuals who practiced mindful eating reported significantly lower cravings for food than the group that did not practice mindfulness.[25] A study in *Cognitive and Behavioral Practice* found "excellent" improvements in symptoms of binge eating in individuals who practiced mindfulness, and these improvements were maintained six months after the mindfulness training had been completed.[26] Researchers from the Oregon Research Institute and the University of New Mexico examined the effects of six weeks of mindful eating training on ten obese patients. After the intervention, the patients lost an average of 9 pounds and lowered their BMIs without making any dietary changes. They also experienced a 39% decrease in hunger, a 60% increase in cognitive restraint (conscious attempts to limit or monitor your food intake), and a 35% decrease in anxiety.[27] If you take the time to enjoy your one daily meal mindfully, you will find it that much more filling, satisfying, and enjoyable.

25 Hugo J. E. M. Alberts, et al., "Coping with Food Cravings. Investigating the Potential of a Mindfulness-Based Intervention," *Appetite* 55, no. 1 (2010): 160–163. doi: 10.1016/j.appet.2010.05.044.

26 Ruth Baer et al., "Mindfulness-Based Cognitive Therapy Applied to Binge Eating: A Case Study," *Cognitive and Behavioral Practice* 12, no. 3 (2005): 351–358.

27 Jeanne Dalen, et al., "Pilot Study: Mindful Eating and Living (MEAL): Weight, Eating Behavior, and Psychological Outcomes Associated with a Mindfulness-Based Intervention for People with Obesity," *Complementary Therapies in Medicine* 18, no. 6 (2010): 260–264. doi: 10.1016/j.ctim.2010.09.008.

Supplements

Apart from the hunger factor making it unsustainable, OMAD detractors might point to the fact that it's impossible to get the recommended daily doses of all the key vitamins and minerals in one meal. That's where supplements come in. If taken carefully and with the knowledge that getting nutrients directly from food is the healthiest route, supplements are a great way to fill the nutritional holes that may occasionally arise from the OMAD diet. What follows are suggestions for types of supplements that may be beneficial, but it is important to talk to a doctor or health care professional regarding doses and formulations.

Multivitamin

Virtually everyone, not just OMAD dieters, could benefit from taking a daily multivitamin. Even people eating a healthy, varied diet may experience minor deficiencies from time to time, so using a multi to make up for those should they arise is a smart choice. What's more, because multivitamins are stuffed with so many different vitamins and minerals, they are typically present in amounts that are easily digested and utilized by the body. This is in contrast to some individual supplements, which might contain more of one vitamin than the body is able to absorb at one time.

As far as choosing a multivitamin, look for one with a seal stating that it has been verified by the United States Pharmacopeial Convention. This seal means that the product contains the ingredients written on the label, does not contain harmful levels of contaminants like pesticides or heavy metals, will break down in your body quickly enough for the ingredients to be absorbed, and has been made according to FDA Good Manufacturing Practices. The amounts of each ingredient should be close to 100% of daily value, with the exception of calcium and magnesium, which would make the pill too big to swallow so will be present in smaller amounts. Higher than 100% is not always better, as some micronutrients can be toxic or simply unable to be utilized at too large amounts. In most cases, multivitamins marketed toward a specific gender or age group tend to be pricier but contain very similar formulas to the same company's regular multivitamin, so in most cases the latter will suffice. And don't be afraid to go for a generic brand: Studies by Consumer Reports have found that store brands test just as highly in terms of formula and dissolution as name brands do but are often a fraction of the price.

These are the vitamins and minerals to look for when selecting a multivitamin:

- Biotin (vitamin B7)
- Calcium
- Folic acid (vitamin B9)
- Iodine
- Iron*
- Magnesium
- Manganese
- Molybdenum
- Niacin (vitamin B3)
- Pantothenic acid (vitamin B5)
- Riboflavin (vitamin B2)
- Selenium
- Thiamin (vitamin B1)
- Vitamin A
- Vitamin B6
- Vitamin B12
- Vitamin C
- Vitamin D3
- Vitamin E
- Vitamin K
- Zinc

*It is important to check with your doctor before taking a supplement that contains iron, as it can be harmful for people in certain age groups or with certain conditions.

Fiber Supplements

For those worried about hunger throughout the day or who favor recipes that don't contain as much fiber, fiber supplements can help. For the maximum satiety-boosting benefits, try a powder that dissolves in liquid and drink it in water or in one of the fast-approved drinks in Chapter 5 whenever you need to throughout the day. A fiber supplement can also help regulate your digestive system and daily bowel movements, which may become irregular when dropping to one meal a day. There are a few common types of fiber supplements. Inulin is a soluble fiber that is also a prebiotic, meaning it feeds the healthy bacteria living in the gut while also helping prolong feelings of fullness. This is crucial because these bacteria impact countless processes, from nutrient absorption to metabolism to hormone production. Another option is psyllium, which is 70% soluble fiber and 30% insoluble fiber, meaning it passes through the gut intact and primarily impacts satiety and digestive regularity.

Omega-3 Supplements

Omega-3 fatty acids, which were mentioned briefly in the section on fats earlier in the chapter, are essential nutrients that the body cannot make by itself. Found in fatty fish, like salmon, mackerel, herring, and tuna, and plant sources like flax seeds, chia seeds, and walnuts, omega-3s play an important role in brain function, inflammation, and healthy growth and development. Deficiencies have been linked to a variety of problems, heart disease among them. For this reason, thousands of people take fish oil supplements. And while fish oil is an often-prescribed and effective treatment for people with high triglyceride levels (which have been linked to heart disease and stroke), the benefits of the supplement for healthy people are still inconclusive. Nonetheless, if you don't eat fish and your doctor or health care practitioner has suggested taking a fish oil supplement, it may help you avoid an omega-3 deficiency. Look for pills that contain both DHA and EPA, the two main omega-3s found in fish.

* * *

If you're conscientious about the foods that make up your one meal a day, choosing foods rich in protein, fiber, and healthy fats and low in sugar and processed carbohydrates, you will have a filling, nourishing, and delicious meal. Eat whenever is most convenient for you to sprinkle in some mindful eating, top things off with smart supplements, and you have the tools to find instant success with the OMAD diet.

CHAPTER 3

What You Can Have During Your Fast

While the premise of the one meal a day diet is to consume all your daily calories at one time, it does not mean that you are forbidden to put anything else in your mouth throughout the day. In fact, there are options for drinking and eating that will not only help you get through the fast happily and painlessly, but can also help optimize your body's slimming systems in order to take full advantage of the eating plan. As a general rule of thumb, you want to avoid eating and drinking things that contain any sugar or carbohydrates, as these will pull your body out of its fasted state and prompt it to use glucose for fuel instead of fat. But as for the things you can enjoy, some of your best options will be listed in this chapter.

Water

Water is your best friend on any diet plan, but especially one that involves extended fasts. One of the reasons that most people don't drink enough water throughout the day is that they often mistake thirst for hunger, finding a snack when a glass of water will suffice. Indeed, water can have a powerful effect on satiety. In one study from 2018, subjects who drank water before a meal consumed up to three times less food during that meal compared to those who did not drink any water prior to eating, suggesting that the water helped them feel fuller faster.[28] Researchers from Virginia Tech found that dieters who drank 500 milliliters, or 16.9 ounces of water (the size of a standard water bottle) prior to each meal showed a 44% greater decline in weight over the 12-week study period.[29] British scientists have found that about 500 milliliters causes enough stretching in the stomach for satiety signals to be sent to the brain.

In addition to helping boost satiety and increase weight loss, water is essential to all of the body's processes. The body of the average adult is about 60% water. It helps transport nutrients and oxygen through the bloodstream to the organs and cells that need them, helps flush out waste and toxins through urination, regulates body temperature through sweat, lubricates joints, and acts as a protective shock absorber for the brain and spinal cord. It is a building block of cells, which are the building blocks of everything in our bodies. The brain is 73% water, and it uses it to build the hormones, neurotransmitters, and other chemical signals that govern every bodily process. The role of water in life and well-being cannot be overlooked.

Average daily water intake in the US is about 39 ounces (or 2⅓ bottles of water), according to the Centers for Disease Control and Prevention, yet the recommendations from the National Academies of Sciences, Engineering, and Medicine are 124 ounces for men, or about 7 bottles of water, and 92 ounces for women, or close to 5½ bottles of water—the closer you get to

28 Ji Na Jeong, "Effect of Pre-meal Water Consumption on Energy Intake and Satiety in Non-obese Young Adults," *Clinical Nutrition Research* 7, no. 4 (2018): 291–296.

29 Elizabeth A. Dennis, et al., "Water Consumption Increases Weight Loss during a Hypocaloric Diet Intervention in Middle-Aged and Older Adults," *Obesity* 18, no. 2 (2010): 300–307.

those numbers, the easier your fast will be. For the purposes of boosting satiety during a fast, sparkling water can also be helpful, provided it is free of sugar and artificial sweeteners. But you don't need to hit these numbers with plain water alone. The drinks that follow, like coffee and tea, can be counted toward your total water intake, helping you hit your goal that much faster.

Coffee

According to the National Coffee Association's annual survey from 2019, 63% of Americans drink at least one cup of coffee per day and 61% of Americans enjoy a daily gourmet coffee beverage, which includes brewed gourmet coffee, espresso-based beverages, and non-espresso-based beverages like blended drinks or cold brew. The good news? Coffee, provided it is consumed a certain way, is a perfect accompaniment to the OMAD diet. Recent studies have shown that coffee has a variety of health benefits, including reducing risk of cardiovascular disease, type 2 diabetes, Parkinson's disease, uterine and liver cancers, cirrhosis, and gout. A 2015 study found that coffee consumption was associated with an 8% to 15% reduction in risk of death, with reductions growing as coffee consumption increased.[30]

Coffee can also be a powerful tool when it comes to losing weight. Coffee contains a potent antioxidant called chlorogenic acid that improves the function of the hormone adiponectin, which facilitates fat burning as well as helps steady blood sugar levels to minimize the surges that signal the body to store fat instead of burning it. According to research published in 2017, subjects who were given the amount of chlorogenic acid in four cups of coffee daily saw a

---

30 Ming Ding, et al., "Association of Coffee Consumption with Total and Cause-Specific Mortality in 3 Large Prospective Cohorts," *Circulation* 132, no. 24 (2015): 2305–2315.

50% increase in the breakdown of stored fat after just 5 days.[31] A separate study from The Netherlands looked at the effects of chlorogenic acid and trigonelline, another plant substance in coffee, on glucose and insulin levels. They found that both glucose and insulin were lower after consumption of these compounds compared with consumption of a placebo.[32]

Here's the catch: If you want to have a cup of hot or iced coffee while on OMAD, it must be black. The exceptions are the coffee-based drinks in Chapter 5, which are mostly blended. But in order to get the most perks out of your fast, your coffee needs to be free of all sugar and artificial sweeteners, as well as any dairy or non-dairy milks and creamers. These add-ins will spike blood sugar and pull the body out of a fat-burning, fasted state. Mix-ins that won't have this effect include coconut oil, unsweetened coconut milk, grass-fed butter, and raw cacao powder (for ways to incorporate these ingredients into your java, check out Chapter 5, beginning on page 60). Coconut oil, unsweetened coconut milk, and grass-fed butter are made up primarily or exclusively of fat, so they won't deter the body from continuing to burn fat (more on this a bit later in the chapter), while raw cacao can provide a chocolaty flavor without any of the sugar or processing in other chocolate products.

Tea

If you know anyone who does not drink coffee, chances are they drink tea. In fact, aside from water, black tea is the most consumed beverage in the world. And like its brewed cousin, tea can be a

31 Insung Park, et al., "Effects of Subacute Ingestion of Chlorogenic Acids on Sleep Architecture and Energy Metabolism through Activity of the Autonomic Nervous System: A Randomized, Placebo-Controlled, Double-Blinded Cross-over Trial," *British Journal of Nutrition* 117, no. 7 (2017): 979–984.

32 Aimee E. Van Dijk, et al., "Acute Effects of Decaffeinated Coffee and the Major Coffee Components Chlorogenic Acid and Trigonelline on Glucose Tolerance," *Diabetes Care* 32, no. 6 (2009): 1023–1025.

boon on an OMAD diet for a few reasons. First, tea has been found to be beneficial for everything from high blood sugar and high cholesterol to heart disease and weight loss. Drinking black tea has been found to reduce triglyceride levels by 36%, blood glucose levels by 18%, and the ratio of LDL cholesterol to HDL cholesterol by 17%.[33] Australian and Dutch researchers reported that regular tea consumption of three cups per day can significantly lower both systolic and diastolic blood pressure (both numbers in your blood pressure reading).[34] And a Swedish study that followed nearly 75,000 people for over 10 years found that those who drank 4 or more cups of tea daily had a 32% lower risk of stroke than those who did not.[35]

Tea also has powerful slimming perks. The primary antioxidant in green tea, EGCG, inhibits the activity of an enzyme that breaks down norepinephrine, a hormone that promotes fat burning in higher concentrations. It has also been found to increase metabolic rate, to the effect of an extra 60 to 160 calories burned per day. In a Japanese study, subjects who drank a beverage containing tea catechins daily saw an 8% increase in calorie burning at rest, a 331% increase in calorie burning during exercise, and a 248% increase in fat burning during exercise.[36]

Because coffee has such a strong flavor on its own, it is difficult to significantly alter that flavor with add-ins that are allowed on the OMAD diet. Tea, on the other hand, can be virtually any flavor you want it to be since those flavor boosters are not being ingested. For

---

33 Theeshan Bahorun, et al., "The Effect of Black Tea on Risk Factors of Cardiovascular Disease in a Normal Population," *Preventive Medicine* 54, supplement (2012): S98–S102.

34 Jonathan M. Hodgson, et al., "Effects of Black Tea on Blood Pressure: A Randomized Controlled Trial," *Archives of Internal Medicine* 172, no. 2 (2012): 186–188.

35 Susanna C. Larsson, et al., "Black Tea Consumption and Risk of Stroke in Women and Men," *Annals of Epidemiology* 23, no. 3 (2013):157–160.

36 Noriyasu Ota, et al., "Effects of Combination of Regular Exercise and Tea Catechins Intake on Energy Expenditure in Humans," *Journal of Health Science* 51, no. 2 (2004): 233–236.

someone with a sweet tooth, hibiscus or dandelion root tea might be the answer. For someone who enjoys an earthier sip, perhaps black or green or even mushroom tea will do the trick. As with coffee, as long as no sweeteners or dairy or nondairy milks are being added, any and all teas are welcome during the fast. Store-bought loose-leaf teas and teabags will certainly do the trick, but Chapter 5 is also filled with homemade teas (beginning on page 64) that use whole fresh herbs and spices like cinnamon sticks, fresh ginger, and vanilla beans to create warm and satisfying brews. When brewing these homemade teas, stick to whole spices over ground ones, as it is impossible to fully strain out ground spices and you could risk a blood sugar spike.

OMAD SUCCESS STORY: MELISSA, 34

In 2017, Melissa began seeing a doctor about what more she could do to help her get pregnant. When the doctor recommended weight loss, Melissa was filled with dread. She had tried countless diets over the years, including Weight Watchers, Beachbody, and only drinking shakes, and the results were always the same: she would lose some weight, but then she would plateau, become discouraged, fall off the plan, and put the pounds back on. But this time there was more at stake. Whatever Melissa did needed to work.

In the spring of 2019, Melissa's doctor recommended a keto diet. She was skeptical but did some research and decided to start it that June. She knew that she needed to lose at least 30 pounds to be able to start her fertility treatments, so she dove in. She lost weight steadily for about two months, but then something familiar happened; she hit a plateau and didn't lose weight for three weeks.

When it came time for her weigh-in to start the treatment, she was still 10 pounds away from her goal, and she wasn't approved.

Returning home discouraged, Melissa began looking online for other options when she came across information on fasting. The thought of trying it made her nervous and she was sure it would sap her energy and make her feel nauseated, but the information she found was compelling enough to give it a try.

The last week of August, Melissa began. She would wake up and have a glass of water, followed by black coffee. At lunchtime she would drink chicken broth, sometimes adding butter to it to make it feel more substantial. She would sip tea and water throughout the day, aiming for 2 to 3 liters total. Then, at dinner, she would eat her one meal, a chicken curry or steak or fish with Brussels sprouts or broccoli.

Melissa lost six pounds that first week and went back to the doctor. Impressed with Melissa's speedy change, the doctor approved her for treatment. Seeing what OMAD could do, Melissa stuck with it, losing almost 10 more pounds that month. To her surprise, she had more energy than before and even more than when she was on keto. What's more, it has helped her recognize her bad eating habits and changed her perspective on eating for the better and healthier. And in August of 2020, one year after discovering OMAD, Melissa welcomed her first child!

Broth

If plain water, coffee, or tea don't feel substantial enough to keep you going throughout a fast, broth may be the answer. While chicken and beef broth will contain a few calories, they contain negligible amounts of carbohydrates and not enough to break your fast and pull your body out of fat-burning mode. For some, the meaty, savory flavor can be more satisfying and feel more like a "meal" than a bottle of water or a cup of tea, while the fact that it is liquid will still serve to stretch out the stomach and force it to send satiety signals to the brain.

What's more, chicken and beef broth (also known as bone broth in today's health and nutrition circles) deliver some impressive slimming benefits. When animal bones are boiled, the collagen inside the bones is released into the water. Most people know collagen as the protein that improves skin elasticity, keeping it looking firm and young, but collagen and its amino acids, including glycine, lysine, and leucine, also play a role in fat burning and maintaining lean muscle mass. The bones themselves deliver nutrients like magnesium and calcium, while bone marrow is rich in iron, zinc, and manganese. In a 2019 study by Korean researchers, subjects who took collagen saw a decrease in body fat percentage and body fat mass without making any other dietary or lifestyle changes, while the subjects who did not receive collagen experienced an increase in both over the study period.[37]

Store-bought broth would work as a drink to enjoy during your fast, and there are a few recipes for homemade chicken and beef broth in Chapter 5 (starting on page 70). But if your family has passed down a recipe or you already have a favorite, either would be sufficient for keeping you satiated outside of your one meal a day.

---

37 Tak Young Jin, et al., "Effect of Oral Ingestion of Low-Molecular Collagen Peptides Derived from Skate (Raja Kenojei) Skin on Body Fat in Overweight Adults: A Randomized, Double-Blind, Placebo-Controlled Trial," *Marine Drugs* 17, no. 3 (March 7, 2019): 157.

Healthy Fat Add-Ons and Fat Bombs

The only option in this chapter that isn't a liquid, certain healthy fats can be consumed without counteracting the benefits of OMAD's 23-hour fast. The reason for this is simple: Since the body is already utilizing fat as energy, consuming more fat is not going to alter that process in any way. Adding healthy fats like coconut oil, grass-fed butter, and unsweetened coconut milk to beverages, like Brain-Boosting Coffee (page 62) or Golden Milk Latte (page 69), will make those sips feel more substantial plus supply a noticeable energy boost upon drinking. But these fats can also be eaten in the form of a sweet treat called a fat bomb. Made from a fat (such as coconut butter, nut butter, or coconut oil), a binder (such as shredded coconut or almond flour), a flavor (like cacao powder, nuts, citrus zest, or spices), and sometimes a tiny amount of sugar-free sweetener (like stevia or monk fruit), these small, indulgent bites can be the perfect way to sate a snack craving on a particularly difficult day of fasting. They are also a genius dessert option for after your one meal and can be enjoyed guilt-free. Fat bomb recipes begin on page 72.

* * *

As is clear from the name, the OMAD diet is about eating just one meal every day. But utilizing drinks and snacks that will not counteract the benefits of the fast—and in most cases, will actually improve them—helps combat many of the common problems and arguments people have against the eating plan. OMAD may seem like an extreme or drastic change, but it does not have to be. The information in this chapter will help make the transition to one meal a day that much more painless and effortless.

CHAPTER 4

Exercising on the OMAD Diet

Exercise is an important part of any healthy lifestyle. It also requires energy. For that reason, it's common to be wary of whether eating one meal a day can sufficiently support an active lifestyle, or whether it is doable for people looking to make specific physical gains such as building muscle or increasing endurance. But before considering those questions, it's important to understand what is happening in the body when you exercise in a fasted state.

As discussed in Chapter 1, fasting helps regulate insulin production. Exercise improves insulin sensitivity, or how much insulin the body requires to regulate blood sugar levels. When people have high insulin sensitivity, they require very little insulin to be produced to maintain low blood sugar. So coupling fasting, which keeps insulin production at low and steady levels, and exercise, which ensures that the body won't need much insulin in the first place, can be an incredibly beneficial combination for folks trying to avoid weight gain or type 2 diabetes.

Fasting has also been found to increase production of human growth hormone, which plays a key role in facilitating muscle growth, improving bone density, and burning fat, some of the main goals of exercise. If your HGH levels are high at the beginning of a workout, the gains made in these areas throughout the session will be that much greater. Not to mention the fact that fat burning has already increased in the absence of sugar to be utilized as fuel. All told, a study published in the *British Journal of Nutrition* found that people who exercised first thing in the morning on an empty stomach burned 20% more fat than those who ate before exercising.[38]

Just as the timing of your one meal a day totally depends on your schedule and personal preferences, exercise can be dependent on those factors as well. Someone who is always hungry after a workout might want to time their session before their meal, while someone who feels nauseous or sluggish when exercising on an empty stomach may want to complete their workout after their meal. Either way, here are some of the best forms of exercise to incorporate into your one meal a day lifestyle in order to see results fast.

Walking

Walking is one of the best forms of exercise you can do, and it is also the easiest to fit into your day. Simply parking farther away from the entrance to the store or taking the stairs instead of the elevator can help you fit in more walking. It is also one of the easiest forms of exercise to do physically, as it is accessible for all ages and fitness levels and is low impact enough for those with certain physical limitations. The health benefits of walking are vast and varied. Walking can improve cardiovascular and pulmonary fitness, strengthen bones, build lean muscle, burn fat, and improve balance.

---

38 Javier T. Gonzalez, et al., "Breakfast and Exercise Contingently Affect Postprandial Metabolism and Energy Balance in Physically Active Males," *British Journal of Nutrition* 110, no. 4 (2013): 721–732.

A study from Harvard University looked at the activity of 32 genes that promote obesity in over 12,000 people and found that the effects of these genes were cut in half in the people who walked for roughly an hour per day.[39] Researchers from the University of Exeter in the UK found that a 15-minute walk can help curb cravings for sweets and even reduce the amount of sweets eaten in a stressful situation.[40] Walking has also been found to ease joint pain, boost immune function, and even lower the risk of developing certain cancers. What's more, many of these benefits will occur even if walking is broken up into 5- or 10-minute sessions over the course of the day as opposed to one continuous 30- to 60-minute walk. If you're unsure of how much exercise you will be able to do in a fasted state, walking is a great starting point.

Interval Training

Also known as HIIT, or high-intensity interval training, this method of exercise has been the subject of much research in recent years. Perfect for those with busy schedules, these short, high-intensity bursts of activity alternated with low-intensity recovery periods have been shown to provide the same increases in metabolism and calorie burning as a longer, moderate-intensity exercise session, plus similar improvements in key health markers like insulin sensitivity and arterial stiffness (a risk factor for heart disease). In a study from Denmark, patients with type 2 diabetes were assigned to either a continuous walking group or an interval walking group. After four months, the subjects in the interval walking group lost 90% more body mass, 98% more fat, and 47% more visceral fat

---

39 Qibin Qi, et al., "Television Watching, Leisure Time Physical Activity, and the General Predisposition in Relation to Body Mass Index in Women and Men," *Circulation* 126, no. 15 (2012): 1821–1827.

40 Hwajung Oh, et al., "Brisk Walking Reduces Ad Libitum Snacking in Regular Chocolate Eaters during a Workplace Simulation," *Appetite* 58, no. 1 (2011): 387–392.

(the dangerous fat that accumulates around the organs) than those in the continuous walking group. Glycemic control, or the patients' abilities to regulate their glucose levels, also improved in the interval walking group.[41]

The high-intensity bursts can take any form, from something challenging cardiovascularly like walking, running, or jumping rope, to something that challenges the muscles, such as squats or push-ups, to movements that combine the two, like burpees. A 10- to 15-minute long HIIT session is enough to reap the benefits, and the lengths of your high-intensity intervals and recovery periods are up to you. If you're new to HIIT and the idea of pushing yourself to your max, start with a 1:3 ratio, or a 20-second burst followed by 1 minute of recovery, repeated 7 times. Then gradually increase the length of your burst or decrease the length of your recovery to challenge yourself even more.

OMAD SUCCESS STORY: ADAM, 27

Adam entered college with hopes of making an immediate impact on his school's basketball team. But at 235 pounds and with well over 20% body fat, he was not in the best shape to do so. Adam had always had a slow metabolism and struggled to gain muscle while easily packing on fat. Up to that point he had never attempted to drastically change his diet, but he knew that if he wanted to achieve his basketball goals, he needed to do something.

Adam headed online to do some research. When he came across the story of former professional football player Herschel Walker, who claimed to only eat one meal a day, he was intrigued. Adam

---

41 Kristian Karstoft, et al., "The Effects of Free-Living Interval-Walking Training on Glycemic Control, Body Composition, and Physical Fitness in Type 2 Diabetic Patients: A Randomized, Controlled Trial," *Diabetes Care* 36, no. 2 (2013): 228–236.

assumed that he would be hungry all day if he was only eating one meal, but as he delved deeper into the science, he became more confident that his body would adapt to the way of eating and he would be fitter and stronger because of it. So he started fasting.

Adam was hungry at first, but that quickly went away, and he began to feel more energetic. He would train first thing in the morning before having his one meal between 12:00 p.m. and 3:00 p.m. At that meal, he would try to fill his plate with 40% protein, 40% healthy fats, and 20% carbs for optimal energy levels. During the rest of the day he sipped tea or coffee blended with coconut oil and cinnamon or drank a branched chain amino acid supplement for additional protein without any carbs or sugar.

Shortly after switching to just one meal a day, Adam began to burn fat and gain muscle. Over his four years of college, his weight increased to 255 pounds, but his body fat percentage dropped to 8%, ideal for an aspiring professional athlete. Fasting has also improved his digestion and even lowered the number of tics he experiences from his Tourette syndrome. In the five years since college, Adam has played professional basketball in Europe and developed his brand, AdamKempFitness.com. He tries to stick to his one meal a day diet as much as he can, as he does not believe he would be where he is today without it.

Strength Training

Strength training, also known as resistance training or simply lifting weights, has become much more mainstream in recent years among exercisers who aren't just trying to bulk up, mainly because the benefits of building muscle for all genders and age groups has become more apparent. Strength training helps build and maintain lean muscle mass, which decreases with age but is critical for maintaining a healthy metabolism and sustaining weight loss. Researchers from Wake Forest University compared the weight loss results of dieters who did not exercise and those who did aerobic exercise to those who completed strength training. They found that the strength trainers lost 80% more weight than the non-exercisers and 13% more weight than the aerobic exercisers. The strength group also lost 12% more fat and 40% less muscle than the aerobics group.[42]

Strong muscles help take pressure off of the joints, lowering the risk of developing arthritis and the instances of joint replacements, plus reduces wear on the bones, helping to maintain healthy bone density. Working with weights, especially if you are in an older age group, helps improve balance, stability, and posture, which can increase mobility. In a 2017 study by the American Society for Bone and Mineral Research, postmenopausal women with low bone density who completed a twice-weekly resistance training regimen saw improvements in functional movements, bone density, and bone strength.[43]

The benefits of strength training are accessible to all ages and fitness levels. Exercises that use your own body weight as resistance, such as push-ups or planks, are perfect for those who don't have access to or don't want to use weights. Resistance bands are easy to use anywhere and can provide a personalized amount of resistance. Weight-training machines can help isolate different muscle groups, while free weights will activate multiple muscle groups at once. The Department of Health and Human Services suggests

---

42 Kristen M. Beavers, et al., "Effects of Exercise Type during Intentional Weight Loss of Body Composition in Older Adults with Obesity," *Obesity* 25, no. 11 (2017): 1823–1829.

43 Steven L. Watson, et al., "High-Intensity Resistance and Impact Training Improves Bone Mineral Density and Physical Function in Postmenopausal Women with Osteopenia and Osteoporosis: The LIFTMOR Randomized Controlled Trial," *Journal of Bone and Mineral Research* 33, no. 2 (2017): 211–220.

incorporating strength training into your exercise routine twice a week, though additional sessions can speed up weight loss.

Fun Movement

Hiking, dancing, cycling, rowing, yoga, Pilates…the list of activities that will deliver the perks of exercise goes on and on, and every single one delivers additional benefits as well. Outdoor activities like hiking and biking come with the stress-reducing perk of being in nature, surrounded by greenery and fresh air. Dancing on your own or in a group class provides a body positivity and self-confidence boost. Yoga works to establish a connection between the mind and the body, which can help reduce stress and anxiety, plus helps improve flexibility and balance.

* * *

In a nutshell, any movement is better than no movement at all, even on the OMAD diet. For the fastest results, try to vary the types of exercise and movements you do throughout the week and listen to how your body responds to each one. Experiment with a strength workout before your one meal one day, then a yoga session after your meal the next, and see how your body reacts. The drinks and snacks in Chapter 5 will come in handy to provide energy for exercising. If your one meal is dinner but you want to work out early in the day, have a cup of black coffee or a Mocha "Latte" (page 63) for an energy boost before your session and then a Coconut Lime Fat Bomb (page 74) and some water afterward to keep you going until mealtime.

Part 2: Recipes

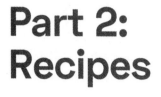

The OMAD diet is incredibly simple: Eat one meal a day. But to get results fast, happily, and without hunger, these recipes are here to help. What follows are 101 recipes that have been specifically formulated to help you stay satiated, energized, and consuming a wide array of nutrients while on the OMAD diet. You'll find drinks and snacks that can be consumed without pulling your body out of its fasting state, followed by tons of recipes for complete, wholesome, hearty meals, like Warm Harissa-Roasted Salmon Salad with Green Beans and Pistachios (page 110), Fall Farro and Chicken Bowl with Roasted Vegetables (page 124), and Grilled Mahi Tacos with Cilantro Lime Rice and Avocado Crema (page 162). Most of the recipes are designed to serve one person but can be easily scaled up if you want to share your meal with your partner or family. Those in the final two chapters, Steaming Chilis and Soups and Hearty Helpings, all serve four or more people. Hearty Helpings is where you'll find some slightly more indulgent but still healthy and filling recipes, like the Beef, Spinach, and Pine Nut Un-Stuffed Shells (page 222), Barbecue Pulled Pork Sandwiches with Tangy Coleslaw (page 224), and Kitchen Sink Enchiladas (page 218).

These recipes do not use complicated techniques or cooking methods or difficult-to-find ingredients. My goal was to get a delicious meal to your plate as quickly and with as little stress as possible, so I shared cooking methods that I use as a home cook to get a tasty and healthy meal on the table on a long and busy day. The notes at the beginning of each recipe offer insights into the recipe's development, ingredient tips, ideas for substitutions, and ways to make the recipe adhere to different eating plans. The recipes are also accompanied by nutritional information to let you know exactly what you are eating. I paid special attention to the protein and fiber content of each recipe in order to achieve maximum satiety.

You will see symbols on some of the recipes to help guide you if you are trying to adapt another eating style to your OMAD diet. Here is what they mean:

K The recipe is keto, or the amount of net carbohydrates (total carbs minus fiber) in the recipe is at or under 30 grams.

P The recipe is paleo, or it is free of grains, dairy, legumes, and sugar. Many recipes can be made paleo with the omission of one or two ingredients. These won't have the symbol but will be noted at the beginning of the recipe.

GF The recipe is completely gluten-free.

PB The ingredients in the recipe are plant-based. Plant-based does not equal vegan, though in most cases it would be easy to make these recipes vegan as well.

I hope you enjoy!

CHAPTER 5

Fast-Approved Drinks and Snacks

Coconut Oil Coffee

Why drink black coffee when you can blend in some coconut oil for an added energy boost? The healthy fat won't raise your blood sugar, so it's the perfect way to make your morning sip more substantial.

MAKES: 1 serving   **TOTAL TIME:** 5 minutes

K, P, GF, PB

12 ounces of your favorite brewed coffee

1 to 2 teaspoons coconut oil

Pour the brewed coffee into a blender and add the coconut oil. Blend until the mixture is frothy and the coconut oil is incorporated. Drink immediately.

Calories: 82 **Fat:** 9g **Carbs:** 0g **Fiber:** 0g **Sugar:** 0g **Protein:** 0g

Brain-Boosting Coffee

This sip is modeled on the popular Bulletproof Coffee, which is made with grass-fed butter and MCT oil. Fans of the drink claim that it delivers energy and mental clarity and boosts satiety.

MAKES: 1 serving   **TOTAL TIME:** 5 minutes

K, P, GF

12 ounces of your favorite brewed coffee

1 tablespoon unsalted, grass-fed butter

2 teaspoons MCT oil or coconut oil

Pour the brewed coffee into a blender and add the butter and oil. Blend until the mixture is frothy and the butter and oil are incorporated. Drink immediately.

Calories: 182 **Fat:** 20g **Carbs:** 0g **Fiber:** 0g **Sugar:** 0g **Protein:** 0g

Mocha "Latte"

Cacao is the rawest form of chocolate, before it is transformed into cocoa powder, chocolate bars, and other treats. It's not too sweet but provides the perfect amount of dark chocolate flavor to balance out the bitterness of the coffee.

MAKES: 1 serving   **TOTAL TIME:** 5 minutes

K, P, GF, PB

12 ounces of your favorite brewed coffee

1 to 2 teaspoons coconut oil

1 teaspoon raw cacao powder, like Navitas Organics

Pour the brewed coffee into a blender and add the coconut oil and raw cacao powder. Blend until the mixture is frothy, the coconut oil is incorporated, and the cacao is dissolved. Drink immediately.

Calories: 90 **Fat:** 9g **Carbs:** 1g **Fiber:** 1g **Sugar:** 0g **Protein:** 1g

Cinnamon-Ginger Tea

Ginger has been found to calm numerous GI woes, including nausea, cramps, and bloating. The added sweetness of cinnamon makes this a delightful, spicy-sweet tea.

MAKES: 1 serving   **TOTAL TIME:** 12 minutes

K, P, GF, PB

3 thin slices fresh ginger

2 cinnamon sticks

2 cups filtered water

1. Add the ginger, cinnamon sticks, and water to a small saucepan. Bring to a boil, then turn the heat to medium and simmer for at least 10 minutes.

2. Strain tea into a mug to remove the cinnamon and ginger, and enjoy.

Calories: 0 **Fat:** 0g **Carbs:** 0g **Fiber:** 0g **Sugar:** 0g **Protein:** 0g

Spicy Chai Tea

Chai tea is delicious hot or iced. If you want to drink it iced, double the spices but use the same amount of water. You can find whole spices at spice stores, some health food stores, or online.

MAKES: 1 serving **TOTAL TIME:** 10 minutes

K, P, GF, PB

6 whole green cardamom pods, smashed

3 thin slices fresh ginger

2 cinnamon sticks

1 teaspoon coriander seeds

1 piece star anise

2 cups filtered water

1 black tea bag

1. Add the cardamom pods, ginger, cinnamon sticks, coriander seeds, star anise, and water to a small saucepan. Bring to a boil.

2. Once the water is boiling, turn the heat to low and add the black tea bag. Simmer for 2 minutes, then turn off the heat and let it steep for 2 minutes more. Discard the tea bag and spices, and enjoy.

Calories: 0 **Fat:** 0g **Carbs:** 0g **Fiber:** 0g **Sugar:** 0g **Protein:** 0g

Vanilla Chai Tea

For those who prefer something sweeter than spicy chai, vanilla chai is the thing. Add a splash of full-fat coconut milk for a creamy sip.

MAKES: 1 serving   **TOTAL TIME:** 10 minutes

K, P, GF, PB

4 whole green cardamom pods, smashed

2 cinnamon sticks

½ teaspoon whole cloves

2 thin slices fresh ginger

1 vanilla bean, cut open

2 cups filtered water

1 black tea bag

1. Add the cardamom pods, cinnamon sticks, cloves, ginger, vanilla bean, and water to a small saucepan. Bring to a boil.

2. Once the water is boiling, turn the heat to low and add the black tea bag. Simmer for 2 minutes, then turn off the heat and let it steep for 2 minutes more. Discard the tea bag and spices, and enjoy.

Calories: 0 Fat: 0g **Carbs:** 0g **Fiber:** 0g **Sugar:** 0g **Protein:** 0g

Orange Black Tea

Citrus goes beautifully with bold, black tea. Feel free to include an extra cinnamon stick or a few drops of liquid stevia for added sweetness.

MAKES: 1 serving   **TOTAL TIME:** 10 minutes

K, P, GF, PB

1 orange rind

2 cinnamon sticks

2 whole green cardamom pods, smashed

2 cups filtered water

1 black tea bag

1. Add the orange rind, cinnamon sticks, cardamom pods, and water to a small saucepan. Bring to a boil.

2. Once the water is boiling, turn the heat to low and add the black tea bag. Simmer for 2 minutes, then turn off the heat and let it steep for 2 minutes more. Discard the tea bag and spices, and enjoy.

Calories: 0 **Fat:** 0g **Carbs:** 0g **Fiber:** 0g **Sugar:** 0g **Protein:** 0g

Ginger Lemongrass Green Tea

This tea is tasty hot but is incredibly refreshing iced. To make it iced, use twice as much ginger and lemongrass and two green tea bags but stick with 2 cups of filtered water.

MAKES: 1 serving   **TOTAL TIME:** 10 minutes

K, P, GF, PB

3 thin slices fresh ginger

2 roughly chopped fresh lemongrass stalks

2 cups filtered water

1 green tea bag

1. Add the ginger, lemongrass, and water to a small saucepan. Bring to a boil.

2. Once the water is boiling, turn the heat to low and add the green tea bag. Simmer for 2 minutes, then turn off the heat and let it steep for 2 minutes more. Discard the tea bag and herbs, and enjoy.

Calories: 0 **Fat:** 0g **Carbs:** 0g **Fiber:** 0g **Sugar:** 0g **Protein:** 0g

Golden Milk Latte

The health benefits of a golden milk latte include reduced inflammation, improved mood, and a stronger immune system, among others. Credit goes to curcumin, the active compound in turmeric. Feel free to add a shot of espresso for a caffeine boost.

MAKES: 1 serving   **TOTAL TIME:** 5 minutes

K, P, GF, PB

- 1 ½ cups unsweetened canned coconut milk
- ½ teaspoon turmeric
- ¼ teaspoon ground ginger
- ¼ teaspoon ground cinnamon
- ½ teaspoon vanilla extract

1. In a small saucepan over medium heat, combine the coconut milk, turmeric, ginger, cinnamon, and vanilla. Whisk until it starts to bubble around the edges and is hot but not boiling.

2. Pour into a mug and enjoy.

Calories: 80 **Fat:** 6g **Carbs:** 5g **Fiber:** 2g **Sugar:** 0g **Protein:** 0g

Chicken Broth

This is my grandmother's chicken soup recipe—it is heartwarming and delicious. Using a variety of chicken bones ensures that you get the maximum amount of nutrients in your broth, while the skin delivers savory flavor.

MAKES: 16 servings   **TOTAL TIME:** 3 hours 20 minutes

K, P, GF, PB

- 1 whole chicken, with skin, cut into pieces
- 4 quarts water
- 1 tablespoon kosher salt
- 4 carrots, peeled and roughly chopped
- 1 parsnip, peeled and roughly chopped
- 2 celery stalks, roughly chopped
- 1 turnip, peeled and roughly chopped
- 1 white onion, roughly chopped
- 2 sprigs fresh dill
- 4 sprigs fresh parsley

1. Place the chicken pieces, water, and salt in a large stockpot. Cover and bring to a boil over high heat.

2. Add the remaining ingredients. Cover, turn the heat to low, and simmer for 3 hours.

3. Strain the stock through a fine strainer and discard the vegetables and herbs. Season with salt to taste. Refrigerate until ready to drink.

Calories: 0 Fat: 0g **Carbs:** 0g **Fiber:** 0g **Sugar:** 0g **Protein:** 0g

Beef Broth

Make sure you use a mix of marrow bones and bones that have some meat on them, like short ribs and oxtail. You can skip the roasting step if you don't have time, but it will make your broth that much more delicious.

MAKES: 16 servings   **TOTAL TIME:** 3 hours 45 minutes

K, P, GF, PB

5 pounds mixed beef bones

3 carrots, peeled and roughly chopped

2 white onions, peeled and roughly chopped

3 celery stalks, roughly chopped

4 quarts water

2 tablespoons apple cider vinegar

1 head garlic, peeled and halved

2 bay leaves

2 tablespoons black peppercorns

2 pieces star anise

2 cinnamon sticks

1 tablespoon kosher salt

1. Preheat the oven to 450°F. Spread the bones, carrots, onions, and celery in a single layer on a large rimmed baking sheet. Roast for 45 minutes, tossing halfway through.

2. Place the bones and veggies in a large stockpot. Add the rest of the ingredients. Bring to a boil over high heat, then cover, turn the heat to low, and simmer for 3 hours.

3. Strain the stock through a fine strainer and discard the bones, vegetables, and herbs. Refrigerate until ready to drink.

Calories: 0 **Fat:** 0g **Carbs:** 0g **Fiber:** 0g **Sugar:** 0g **Protein:** 0g

Chocolate Fat Bombs

Fat bombs may not sound appetizing, but these treats taste like thick, rich dark chocolate. One is all you need to satisfy midafternoon cravings.

MAKES: 12 to 16 servings   **TOTAL TIME:** 10 minutes

K, P, GF, PB

½ cup coconut butter, like Artisana

¼ cup raw cacao powder

¼ cup melted coconut oil

2 teaspoons liquid stevia

1. In a bowl, stir together all of the ingredients until smooth.

2. Spoon the mixture into a muffin tin or an ice cube tray and freeze until set. Store in the freezer.

Calories: 135 **Fat:** 13g **Carbs:** 6g **Fiber:** 4g **Sugar:** 1g **Protein:** 2g

Almond Fat Bombs

The combination of almond butter and almond extract makes for a pronounced nutty flavor. Both unsalted and salted almond butter are tasty, but use a natural one without any other added ingredients.

MAKES: 12 to 16 servings   **TOTAL TIME:** 10 minutes

K, P, GF, PB

½ cup raw almond butter

¼ cup melted coconut oil

2 teaspoons liquid stevia

8 drops almond extract (a little under ¼ teaspoon)

1. In a bowl, stir together all of the ingredients until smooth.

2. Spoon the mixture into a muffin tin or an ice cube tray and freeze until set. Store in the freezer.

Calories: 126 **Fat:** 12g **Carbs:** 4g **Fiber:** 2g **Sugar:** 2g **Protein:** 3g

Coconut Lime Fat Bombs

These have a lovely, zesty, tropical flavor. You can use finely shredded coconut or coconut flakes, as long as they are unsweetened.

MAKES: 12 to 16 servings   **TOTAL TIME:** 10 minutes

K, P, GF, PB

½ cup coconut butter, like Artisana

¼ cup melted coconut oil

¼ cup unsweetened shredded coconut

zest of 2 limes

1 teaspoon liquid stevia

1. In a bowl, stir together all of the ingredients until smooth.

2. Spoon the mixture into a muffin tin or an ice cube tray and freeze until set. Store in the freezer.

Calories: 150 **Fat:** 15g **Carbs:** 5g **Fiber:** 3g **Sugar:** 1g **Protein:** 1g

Chocolate Mint Fat Bombs

A snack that tastes like a York Peppermint Pattie, but healthy? Yes, please!

MAKES: 12 to 16 servings   **TOTAL TIME:** 10 minutes

K, P, GF, PB

½ cup coconut butter, like Artisana

¼ cup raw cacao powder

¼ cup melted coconut oil

2 teaspoons liquid stevia

½ teaspoon peppermint extract

1. In a bowl, stir together all of the ingredients until smooth.

2. Spoon the mixture into a muffin tin or an ice cube tray and freeze until set. Store in the freezer.

Calories: 137 **Fat:** 14g **Carbs:** 6g **Fiber:** 4g **Sugar:** 1g **Protein:** 2g

Gingerbread Fat Bombs

Cashew butter has a subtler flavor than almond butter so the fall spices will stand out more. But if you can't find it, almond butter will work as well.

MAKES: 12 to 16 servings **TOTAL TIME:** 10 minutes

K, P, GF, PB

½ cup almond or cashew butter

¼ cup almond flour or unsweetened shredded coconut

¼ cup melted coconut oil

½ teaspoon ground ginger

¼ teaspoon ground cinnamon

¼ teaspoon ground nutmeg

1 teaspoon liquid stevia

1. In a bowl, stir together all of the ingredients until smooth.

2. Spoon the mixture into a muffin tin or an ice cube tray and freeze until set. Store in the freezer.

Calories: 35 **Fat:** 4g **Carbs:** 0g **Fiber:** 0g **Sugar:** 0g **Protein:** 0g

Vanilla Fat Bombs

These bites deliver smooth, classic vanilla goodness with a hint of coconut.

MAKES: 12 to 16 servings   **TOTAL TIME:** 10 minutes

K, P, GF, PB

½ cup coconut butter, like Artisana

¼ cup melted coconut oil

¼ cup unsweetened shredded coconut

1 teaspoon vanilla extract

1 teaspoon liquid stevia

1. In a bowl, stir together all of the ingredients until smooth.

2. Spoon the mixture into a muffin tin or an ice cube tray and freeze until set. Store in the freezer.

Calories: 155 **Fat:** 15g **Carbs:** 5g **Fiber:** 3g **Sugar:** 1g **Protein:** 1g

CHAPTER 6

Breakfast-Style Meals

Mediterranean Frittata

You can buy feta already crumbled, but it is much creamier and more flavorful if you buy a block and crumble it yourself. Enjoy this frittata with some whole wheat toast for additional fiber.

MAKES: 1 serving   **TOTAL TIME:** 30 minutes

K, GF

1 tablespoon olive oil

½ sweet onion, sliced

½ cup sliced roasted red peppers

¼ cup sliced banana peppers

¼ cup sliced sun-dried tomatoes

1 cup fresh baby spinach

1 small clove garlic, minced

¼ teaspoon dried thyme

pinch of salt

pinch of pepper

6 large eggs

½ cup crumbled feta cheese

1. Preheat the oven to 400°F. Spray a large ovenproof skillet with cooking spray, then add the olive oil and heat over medium heat. Add the onion and cook until soft, about 8 minutes. Add the remaining veggies, garlic, thyme, salt, and pepper. Cook for 2 minutes more, or until the spinach is mostly wilted.

2. In a bowl, whisk together the eggs and crumbled feta. Slowly pour the egg mixture into the pan and use a spatula to gently disperse the filling evenly through the egg.

3. Cook until the edges are just set, about 1 minute. Transfer the pan to the oven and bake until the edges start to brown and the center is set, about 15 minutes.

4. Cool slightly in the pan, then slide it onto a plate and serve.

Calories: 849 **Fat:** 61g **Carbs:** 28g **Fiber:** 5g **Sugar:** 19g **Protein:** 53g

Ham, Cheese, and Veggie Frittata

I don't love the texture of tomatoes in eggs but using them as a garnish brings brightness and freshness to this frittata. Enjoy it with a slice of whole grain toast for additional fiber and skip the cheese to make this meal paleo.

MAKES: 1 serving   **TOTAL TIME:** 30 minutes

GF

1 tablespoon olive oil

1 medium yellow onion, chopped

1 green bell pepper, chopped

1 large russet potato, peeled (if desired) and chopped

1 cup chopped cooked ham

pinch of salt

pinch of pepper

6 large eggs

1 cup shredded cheddar cheese

½ cup diced tomatoes or pico de gallo

1. Preheat the oven to 400°F. Spray a large ovenproof skillet with cooking spray, then add the olive oil and heat over medium heat. Add the onion, green bell pepper, and potato, and cook until soft, about 10 minutes. Add the ham, salt and pepper, and toss to combine.

2. In a bowl, whisk together the eggs and shredded cheddar. Slowly pour the egg mixture into the pan and use a spatula to gently disperse the filling evenly through the egg.

3. Cook until the edges are just set, about 1 minute. Transfer the pan to the oven and bake until the edges start to brown and the center is set, about 15 minutes.

4. Cool slightly in the pan, then loosen with the spatula and slide onto a plate. Top with the diced tomatoes or pico de gallo, and serve.

Calories: 1,454 **Fat:** 94g **Carbs:** 61g **Fiber:** 11g **Sugar:** 17g **Protein:** 95g

Frittata Primavera

Feel free to sub in any of your favorite vegetables that aren't present or skip the cheese to make it paleo.

MAKES: 1 serving   **TOTAL TIME:** 30 minutes

K, GF

1 tablespoon olive oil

½ cup diced asparagus

¼ cup diced zucchini

¼ cup diced yellow squash

½ cup chopped broccoli

¼ cup peas, fresh or frozen

1 cup fresh baby spinach

pinch of salt

pinch of pepper

6 large eggs

1 cup shredded mozzarella cheese

2 tablespoons grated Parmesan cheese

1. Preheat the oven to 400°F. Spray a large ovenproof skillet with cooking spray, then add the olive oil and heat over medium heat. Add the asparagus, zucchini, squash, broccoli, and peas, and cook for 8 minutes. Add the spinach, salt, and pepper, and cook for 2 minutes more, or until the spinach is mostly wilted.

2. In a bowl, whisk together the eggs and mozzarella. Slowly pour the egg mixture into the pan and use a spatula to gently disperse the filling evenly. Sprinkle with the grated Parmesan.

3. Cook until the edges are just set, about 1 minute. Transfer the pan to the oven and bake until the edges start to brown and the center is set, about 15 minutes.

4. Cool slightly in the pan. Loosen with a spatula to slide it onto a plate and serve.

Calories: 773 **Fat:** 51g **Carbs:** 26g **Fiber:** 9g **Sugar:** 11g **Protein:** 57g

Acai-Berry Smoothie Bowl

Sweet acai berries are one of the most antioxidant-rich foods in the world. Check the freezer aisle in your grocery store for packs of the frozen berry puree. This bowl will be gluten-free if you omit the granola and plant-based if you use plant-based (like coconut or cashew) yogurt and protein powder.

MAKES: 1 serving   **TOTAL TIME:** 10 minutes

1 (3.5-ounce) frozen unsweetened acai puree pack, like Sambazon

½ cup fresh blueberries, divided

½ cup fresh raspberries, divided

½ cup plain or vanilla Greek yogurt

2 scoops of your favorite protein powder

1 cup fresh baby spinach

½ avocado, peeled and pitted

1 tablespoon chia seeds

¼ cup unsweetened coconut flakes

¼ cup fruit and nut granola

1 banana, sliced

1. Place the acai puree, half the blueberries and raspberries, the yogurt, protein powder, spinach, and avocado in a blender and blend until smooth. Scoop into a bowl.

2. Top the smoothie mixture with the remaining berries, chia seeds, coconut flakes, granola, and banana, and serve.

Calories: 1,275 **Fat:** 83g **Carbs:** 121g **Fiber:** 39g **Sugar:** 47g **Protein:** 76g

Tropical Smoothie Bowl

Mango does not have a lot of water in it, so this smoothie bowl is super thick and creamy. The combination of mango, pineapple, banana, and coconut will transport you to your favorite beach. Use plant-based yogurt and protein powder to make this bowl plant-based.

MAKES: 1 serving   **TOTAL TIME:** 10 minutes

GF

1 cup frozen mango chunks

1 cup frozen pineapple chunks

1 frozen banana

½ cup coconut-flavored Greek yogurt

½ cup coconut water, plus more if needed

2 scoops of your favorite protein powder

1 cup fresh baby spinach

½ avocado, peeled and pitted

1 tablespoon flax seeds

¼ cup unsweetened coconut flakes

1 kiwi, sliced

¼ cup fresh blueberries

1. Place the mango, pineapple, banana, yogurt, coconut water, protein powder, spinach, and avocado in a blender and blend until smooth, adding more coconut water as needed if the mixture is too thick. Scoop into a bowl.

2. Top the smoothie mixture with the flax seeds, coconut flakes, sliced kiwi, and blueberries, and serve.

Calories: 1,127 **Fat:** 37g **Carbs:** 156g **Fiber:** 23g **Sugar:** 113g **Protein:** 60g

Chocolate-Covered Strawberry Smoothie Bowl

This bowl is a protein- and fiber-rich meal disguised as a sweet, creamy, decadent dessert. Use plant-based yogurt and protein powder to make this bowl plant-based.

MAKES: 1 serving   **TOTAL TIME:** 10 minutes

GF

2 cups frozen strawberries

1 frozen banana

½ cup plain or strawberry Greek yogurt

2 tablespoons cacao powder, like Navitas Organics

2 scoops of your favorite unflavored or chocolate protein powder

1 cup fresh baby spinach

½ avocado, peeled and pitted

1 tablespoon chia seeds

¼ cup sliced almonds

¼ cup sliced fresh strawberries

1. Place the frozen strawberries, banana, yogurt, cacao powder, protein powder, spinach, and avocado in a blender and blend until smooth. Scoop into a bowl.

2. Top the smoothie mixture with the chia seeds, sliced almonds, and sliced fresh strawberries, and serve.

Calories: 990 **Fat:** 48g **Carbs:** 101g **Fiber:** 37g **Sugar:** 36g **Protein:** 72g

Chocolate Almond Loaded Oatmeal

Mixing protein powder into oatmeal is an easy way to up the protein of your meal—make sure to stir it into the hot oatmeal immediately so it dissolves completely. Use almond milk and plant-based protein powder to make the meal plant-based.

MAKES: 1 serving   **TOTAL TIME:** 10 minutes

GF

1 cup regular or almond milk

½ cup old-fashioned oats

1 scoop of your favorite chocolate or unflavored protein powder

2 tablespoons almond or peanut butter

¼ teaspoon ground cinnamon

¼ cup sliced almonds

1 banana, sliced

2 tablespoons chocolate chips

1 tablespoon flax seeds

1. Bring the milk just to a boil in a small saucepan. Stir in the oats, lower the heat to medium, and cook until all the milk is absorbed, 5 to 6 minutes, stirring occasionally.

2. Spoon the oats into a bowl. Stir in the protein powder, almond butter, and cinnamon, then top with the sliced almonds, banana, chocolate chips, and flax seeds. Serve immediately.

Calories: 932 Fat: 50g **Carbs:** 82g **Fiber:** 15g **Sugar:** 42g **Protein:** 49g

Apple Cinnamon Loaded Oatmeal

Feel free to sub in pumpkin pie spice for the nutmeg, if you have it. Use almond milk and plant-based protein powder to make the meal plant-based.

MAKES: 1 serving   **TOTAL TIME:** 10 minutes

GF

1 cup regular or almond milk

½ cup old-fashioned oats

1 apple, peeled (if desired) and diced

½ teaspoon ground cinnamon

pinch of ground nutmeg

1 scoop of your favorite unflavored protein powder

¼ cup chopped pecans

¼ cup raisins

1 tablespoon flax seeds

1 teaspoon raw honey

1. Bring the milk just to a boil in a medium saucepan. Add the oats, apple, cinnamon, and nutmeg and lower the heat to medium. Cook until the milk is absorbed and the apples are soft, about 6 minutes, stirring occasionally.

2. Spoon the oats and apples into a bowl and stir in the protein powder. Top with the chopped pecans, raisins, and flax seeds, and drizzle with the honey. Serve immediately.

Calories: 708 **Fat:** 22g **Carbs:** 103g **Fiber:** 16g **Sugar:** 63g **Protein:** 39g

Pumpkin Spice Loaded Oatmeal

This hearty bowl of oatmeal goes all-in on fall with pumpkin pie spice, maple syrup and pumpkin puree, which makes the oatmeal smoother and creamier.

MAKES: 1 serving   **TOTAL TIME:** 10 minutes

GF

- 1 cup regular or almond milk
- ½ cup old-fashioned oats
- ½ cup pumpkin puree
- ½ teaspoon pumpkin pie spice
- 1 scoop of your favorite unflavored protein powder
- ¼ cup chopped walnuts or pecans
- 1 tablespoon flax seeds
- 1 teaspoon maple syrup

1. Bring the milk just to a boil in a medium saucepan. Add the oats, pumpkin puree, and pumpkin pie spice, and lower the heat to medium. Cook until the milk is absorbed, about 6 minutes, stirring occasionally.

2. Spoon the oatmeal into a bowl and stir in the protein powder. Top with the chopped nuts and flax seeds, drizzle with the maple syrup, and serve.

Calories: 712 **Fat:** 36g **Carbs:** 56g **Fiber:** 15g **Sugar:** 21g **Protein:** 48g

Meat-Free Mexican Breakfast Burrito

Before rolling up your burrito, microwave the tortilla for 25 seconds to make it a bit more pliable.

MAKES: 1 serving   **TOTAL TIME:** 15 minutes

1 tablespoon olive oil

½ red or orange bell pepper, chopped

¼ white or sweet onion, chopped

1 medium red bliss potato, peeled (if desired) and chopped

5 large eggs

¼ cup heavy cream

¼ cup canned black beans, drained and rinsed

¼ cup shredded cheddar or Mexican blend cheese

1 large whole wheat tortilla

¼ cup prepared salsa

1. In a skillet over medium-high heat, heat the olive oil. Add the bell pepper, onion, and potato, and cook until everything is soft and cooked through, about 10 minutes.

2. In a bowl, whisk together the eggs and cream. Turn the heat on the skillet to medium-low and add the eggs. Cook, stirring with a rubber spatula, until the eggs are fluffy and scrambled, about 4 minutes.

3. Turn off the heat but don't move the skillet. Add the beans and cheese, stir to combine, and let it sit for a minute or so while the cheese melts.

4. Place the large tortilla on a plate. Transfer the egg mixture to the tortilla and top with the salsa. Roll it up and serve warm.

Calories: 1,073 **Fat:** 61g **Carbs:** 84g **Fiber:** 14g **Sugar:** 10g **Protein:** 53g

Farmer's Market Breakfast Burrito

Spreading fresh spinach on the tortilla before topping with the avocado and egg mixture gives this burrito some crunch alongside the soft and creamy scramble.

MAKES: 1 serving   **TOTAL TIME:** 15 minutes

K

1 tablespoon olive oil

¼ white or sweet onion, chopped

½ cup broccoli florets

¼ cup diced asparagus

¼ cup diced white mushrooms

5 large eggs

¼ cup heavy cream

¼ cup shredded Swiss or mozzarella cheese

1 large whole wheat tortilla

½ cup fresh spinach leaves

½ avocado, peeled, pitted, and sliced thin

1. In a skillet over medium-high heat, heat the olive oil. Add the onion, broccoli, asparagus, and mushrooms, and cook until everything is soft and cooked through, about 8 minutes.

2. In a bowl, whisk together the eggs and cream. Turn the heat on the skillet to medium-low and add the eggs. Cook, stirring with a rubber spatula, until the eggs are fluffy and scrambled, about 4 minutes.

3. Turn off the heat but don't move the skillet. Add the cheese, stir to combine, and let it sit for a minute or so while the cheese melts.

4. Place the large tortilla on a plate. Spread the fresh spinach on the tortilla, followed by the sliced avocado. Top with the egg mixture, roll it up, and serve warm.

Calories: 956 **Fat:** 72g **Carbs:** 42g **Fiber:** 13g **Sugar:** 5g **Protein:** 43g

Veggie Scramble Skillet

Sure, you may not own an adorable mini cast-iron skillet like the one at your favorite breakfast spot, but you can make an equally delicious breakfast skillet at home. Add some whole wheat toast for added fiber. And if you do have a mini skillet, even better!

MAKES: 1 serving   **TOTAL TIME:** 25 minutes

K, GF

1 cup frozen tater tots	salt, to taste
1 tablespoon olive oil	pepper, to taste
¼ cup broccoli florets	1 cup fresh baby spinach
¼ sweet onion, chopped	4 large eggs
¼ red bell pepper, chopped	¼ cup heavy cream
¼ cup chopped white mushrooms	¼ cup shredded cheese, like mozzarella or Swiss

1. Cook the tater tots according to the package instructions.

2. Heat the olive oil in a skillet over medium heat. Add the broccoli, onion, bell pepper, and mushrooms. Season with salt and pepper, and cook until soft, about 8 minutes. Add the spinach and toss until it begins to wilt, about 1 minute.

3. In a bowl, whisk together the eggs and cream. Turn the heat to medium-low and pour the eggs over the veggies. Cook until softly scrambled, about 3 minutes.

4. When the tater tots are done, add them to the skillet with the eggs and veggies.

5. Sprinkle the cheese over everything. Turn off the heat, lay a piece of aluminum foil over the pan, and let the cheese melt for a few minutes. Slide everything onto a plate and serve.

Calories: 757 **Fat:** 55g **Carbs:** 31g **Fiber:** 4g **Sugar:** 6g **Protein:** 37g

Meat Lover's Skillet

Perhaps you prefer home fries and meat to tater tots and veggies. If so, give this skillet a try!

MAKES: 1 serving   **TOTAL TIME:** 25 minutes

GF

1 large Yukon Gold potato, diced

3 slices bacon

1 link or 2 patties breakfast sausage

½ white onion, chopped

salt, to taste

pepper, to taste

4 large eggs

¼ cup heavy cream

¼ cup shredded cheddar cheese

1. Place the diced potatoes in a small pot. Cover them with cold water, bring to a boil over high heat, and boil for 5 minutes. Drain well.

2. Meanwhile, heat a skillet over medium heat. Add the bacon and cook, turning, until it reaches your desired crispiness, about 5 minutes total. Use tongs to remove the bacon to a paper towel–lined plate, leaving the bacon fat in the pan. Let it cool slightly and then chop.

3. Add the sausage and onion to the skillet and cook, breaking up the sausage, until it is cooked through and the onions are soft, about 6 minutes. Remove and set aside.

4. Spread the diced potatoes in a single layer in the pan. Season with salt and pepper and cook them for 3 minutes without disturbing them so they can brown. Toss them around and cook about 3 minutes more to brown the other sides.

5. Return the bacon, sausage, and onions to the pan and turn the heat to medium-low. In a bowl, whisk together the eggs and cream, and pour them over the veggies. Cook until softly scrambled, about 3 minutes.

6. Sprinkle the cheese over everything. Turn off the heat, lay a piece of aluminum foil over the pan, and let the cheese melt for a few minutes. Slide everything onto a plate and serve.

Calories: 1,186 **Fat:** 66g **Carbs:** 79g **Fiber:** 9g **Sugar:** 9g **Protein:** 72g

CHAPTER 7

Giant Salads

Greek Steak Tip Salad

There's a takeout joint in my hometown known mostly for its roast beef and Greek pizza, but to me it will always be the steak tip salad place. This spin on that salad is fresh and delicious. Skip the feta to make it paleo.

MAKES: 1 serving **TOTAL TIME:** 20 minutes

K, GF

6 ounces steak tips or sirloin steak, cut into chunks

2 teaspoons red wine vinegar

2 teaspoons lemon juice

2 tablespoons olive oil

1 small clove garlic, minced

¼ teaspoon dried oregano

¼ teaspoon salt, plus more for steak

⅛ teaspoon pepper, plus more for steak

½ cucumber, sliced

½ cup cherry tomatoes, halved

¼ cup black olives, sliced

¼ red onion, thinly sliced

¼ cup crumbled feta cheese

¼ cup shelled pistachios

1 tablespoon flax seeds

3 cups mixed greens

1. Heat a grill or grill pan over medium heat and grease with cooking spray. Season the steak tips with salt and pepper. Cook, turning, 8 minutes for medium or to desired doneness.

2. In a bowl, whisk together the red wine vinegar, lemon juice, olive oil, garlic, oregano, ¼ teaspoon of salt, and ⅛ teaspoon of pepper.

3. In a large bowl, combine the cucumber, tomatoes, olives, onion, feta, pistachios, flax seeds, and greens. Top with the steak tips, drizzle with the dressing, and serve.

Calories: 981 **Fat:** 63g **Carbs:** 37g **Fiber:** 15g **Sugar:** 8g **Protein:** 70g

Roasted Vegetable Salad with Grilled Chicken and Goat Cheese

I love the combination of fresh, crisp greens and warm, roasted veggies. Skip the goat cheese to make this salad paleo.

MAKES: 1 serving   **TOTAL TIME:** 45 minutes

K, GF

½ small zucchini, quartered lengthwise

½ bell pepper, stemmed, seeded, and sliced

½ cup broccoli florets

½ cup Brussels sprouts, trimmed and halved

4 tablespoons olive oil, divided

2 small cloves garlic, minced, divided

1 teaspoon dried thyme

6 ounces boneless, skinless chicken breast

1 tablespoon fresh lemon juice

3 cups mixed greens

¼ cup crumbled goat cheese

2 tablespoons chopped walnuts

salt and pepper

1. Preheat the oven to 400°F. Cut the zucchini into 1-inch strips. Place them in a bowl with the bell pepper, broccoli, and Brussels sprouts. Add 1 tablespoon olive oil, 1 clove of minced garlic, thyme, salt, and pepper, and toss to coat. Spread in a single layer on a rimmed baking sheet and roast until tender, 20 to 25 minutes.

2. Heat a griddle or grill pan over medium heat. Season the chicken with salt and pepper and grill until cooked through, 6 to 7 minutes per side.

3. In a small bowl, whisk together the remaining olive oil, remaining garlic, lemon juice, and a pinch of salt and pepper.

4. Slice the chicken breast into strips. Place the mixed greens in a large bowl. Top them with the roasted veggies, chicken, goat cheese, and walnuts. Drizzle with the dressing and serve.

Calories: 1,022 **Fat:** 80g **Carbs:** 28g **Fiber:** 9g **Sugar:** 7g **Protein:** 56g

---

Super Cobb with Green Goddess Dressing

I find green goddess dressing to have an incredibly indulgent taste, especially on a salad as savory as a cobb. If you're near a Trader Joe's, they sell a great one made with all-natural ingredients.

MAKES: 1 serving   **TOTAL TIME:** 30 minutes

K, GF

3 slices bacon

2 eggs

6 ounces boneless, skinless chicken breast

salt, to taste

pepper, to taste

2 tablespoons mayonnaise

2 tablespoons plain Greek yogurt

⅓ teaspoon anchovy paste

½ small clove garlic, chopped

2 tablespoons chopped fresh parsley

2 teaspoons chopped fresh tarragon

½ tablespoon chopped chives

1 teaspoon lemon juice

3 cups romaine lettuce

½ cup halved cherry tomatoes

½ cup diced cucumber

¼ cup sliced red onion

¼ cup crumbled blue cheese

½ avocado, peeled, pitted, and sliced

1. Heat a skillet over medium heat. Add the bacon and cook, turning every 2 minutes, until crispy, about 6 minutes. Remove the bacon to a paper towel–lined plate, leaving the bacon fat in the pan. Once the bacon is cool, transfer it to a cutting board and chop.

2. Place the eggs in a small pot and cover them with water. Bring the water to a boil over high heat and boil for 12 minutes. Remove the eggs, run them under cold water, peel away the shells, and chop.

3. Season the chicken breast with salt and pepper then add it to the skillet with the bacon fat. Cook over medium heat until cooked through, about 7 minutes per side. Transfer to a cutting board and cut into cubes.

4. In a blender or food processor, combine the mayo, yogurt, anchovy paste, garlic, parsley, tarragon, chives, and lemon juice, and blend until smooth and creamy.

5. Place the lettuce in a large bowl. Top with the bacon, chicken, hard-boiled eggs, cherry tomatoes, diced cucumber, sliced onion, crumbled blue cheese, and sliced avocado, arranging each ingredient in a row if you're feeling fancy. Drizzle with the green goddess dressing and serve.

Calories: 1,158 **Fat:** 80g **Carbs:** 34g **Fiber:** 10g **Sugar:** 10g **Protein:** 84g

Salmon and Strawberry Salad

This is based on one of my mom's favorite homemade salad recipes. The dressing is a bit of a splurge, but it goes beautifully with the salmon and strawberries.

MAKES: 1 serving   **TOTAL TIME:** 20 minutes

GF

2 tablespoons plus
2 teaspoons olive oil

1 (8-ounce) salmon fillet

salt, to taste

¼ cup slivered almonds

2 tablespoons sugar

2 tablespoons apple
cider vinegar

1 small dash
Worcestershire sauce

½ tablespoon minced onion

2 tablespoons grated
Parmesan cheese

5 ounces fresh baby spinach

1 cup thinly sliced
fresh strawberries

½ cup thinly sliced red onion

¼ cup crumbled goat cheese

1. Heat 2 teaspoons of olive oil in a skillet over medium-high heat. Pat the salmon dry with paper towels and season with salt.

2. Place the salmon in the pan and cook 7 to 9 minutes, or until the light pink color is about ¾ of the way up the fillet. Flip and cook 2 minutes more or to your desired doneness, then transfer to a plate.

3. Spread the slivered almonds on a small baking sheet or toaster oven tray. Heat the oven or toaster oven to 350°F. Add the almonds and toast (checking often, as these can burn very quickly) until the edges are just beginning to brown, about 3 minutes.

4. In a salad dressing cruet or a small bowl, combine the sugar, olive oil, apple cider vinegar, Worcestershire sauce, minced onion, and grated Parmesan. Shake or whisk well, until the sugar is dissolved.

5. Place the spinach in a large bowl. Top with the strawberries, red onion, goat cheese, almonds, and salmon. Drizzle with the dressing and serve.

Calories: 1,105 **Fat:** 76g **Carbs:** 52g **Fiber:** 10g **Sugar:** 36g **Protein:** 66g

Mexican Salad with Corn and Avocado

Be sure to use nonfat yogurt for the dressing, as 2% and whole milk yogurt will be too thick to drizzle.

MAKES: 1 serving   **TOTAL TIME:** 20 minutes

GF

6 ounces boneless skinless turkey breast

¼ teaspoon chili powder

¼ teaspoon ground cumin

¼ cup plain nonfat Greek yogurt

1 teaspoon chipotle in adobo

squeeze of fresh lime juice

salt, to taste

pepper, to taste

3 cups romaine lettuce

1 small tomato, seeded and diced

½ cup frozen corn, thawed

½ cup canned black beans, drained and rinsed

½ avocado, peeled, pitted, and diced

¼ cup shredded Mexican cheese

¼ cup crushed tortilla chips

1. Heat a griddle or grill pan over medium heat. Rub the turkey with the chili powder and cumin. Grill until cooked through, 6 to 7 minutes per side. Cool slightly then cut into strips.

2. In a small bowl, whisk together the Greek yogurt, chipotle sauce, and fresh lime juice. Season to taste with salt and pepper. If it is not thin enough to drizzle, add a little more lime juice.

3. Put the lettuce in a large bowl. Top with the chicken, tomato, corn, black beans, avocado, cheese, and tortilla chips. Drizzle with the creamy chipotle dressing and serve.

Calories: 1,114 **Fat:** 43g **Carbs:** 118g **Fiber:** 27g **Sugar:** 18g **Protein:** 73g

---

Thai Salmon Salad with Coconut Flakes

If you're wary about putting coconut on a salad, don't be! It pairs great with the creamy peanut dressing.

MAKES: 1 serving **TOTAL TIME:** 45 minutes

GF

½ sweet potato, peeled and cut into 1-inch cubes

3 teaspoons olive oil, divided

1 (8-ounce) salmon fillet

salt, to taste

2 tablespoons unsweetened coconut flakes

2 tablespoons chopped peanuts

2 tablespoons creamy peanut butter

1 tablespoon rice or white vinegar

½ tablespoon soy sauce

1 teaspoon honey

pinch of ground ginger

warm water, if needed

½ cucumber, sliced thin

¼ red onion, sliced thin

1 carrot, peeled and shredded

3 cups mixed greens

1. Preheat the oven to 350°F. Toss the sweet potato with 1 teaspoon of olive oil and spread on a small baking sheet. Roast for 25 minutes, or until soft. Remove and set aside but leave the oven on.

2. Heat 2 teaspoons of olive oil in a skillet over medium-high heat. Pat the salmon dry with paper towels and season with salt.

3. Place the salmon in the pan skin-side down and cook 7 to 9 minutes, or until the light pink color is about ¾ of the way up the fillet. Flip and cook 2 minutes more or to your desired doneness, then transfer to a plate.

4. Spread the coconut flakes and chopped peanuts on a small baking sheet. Toast in the oven (checking often, as these can burn very quickly) until the edges are just beginning to brown, about 3 minutes.

5. In a food processor, combine the peanut butter, vinegar, soy sauce, honey, and ginger. Blitz until smooth, adding water as needed, 1 tablespoon at a time, if the dressing is too thick.

6. Place the cucumber, onion, carrot, and greens in a large bowl. Top with the roasted sweet potatoes, salmon, and toasted coconut and peanuts. Drizzle with the peanut dressing and serve.

Calories: 892 **Fat:** 53g **Carbs:** 52g **Fiber:** 12g **Sugar:** 20g **Protein:** 64g

The Triple Chick with Creamy Parmesan Dressing

What is the triple chick? It's chicken, chickpeas, and egg. (Yes, I know that chickpeas don't come from chickens. But it's still in the name.)

MAKES: 1 serving   **TOTAL TIME:** 20 minutes

GF

1 (6-ounce) boneless, skinless chicken breast

salt, to taste

pepper, to taste

1 egg

¼ cup mayonnaise

2 tablespoons grated Parmesan cheese

2 teaspoons fresh lemon juice

1 small clove garlic, minced

½ teaspoon Worcestershire sauce

½ teaspoon Dijon mustard

½ cup sliced roasted red peppers

¼ cup canned chickpeas, drained and rinsed

2 tablespoons flax seeds

½ cup halved cherry tomatoes

¼ cup shaved Parmesan cheese

3 cups baby kale

1. Heat a grill or grill pan over medium heat. Season the chicken with salt and pepper and grill until cooked through, 6 to 7 minutes per side depending on thickness. Let it cool slightly then cut into strips.

2. Place the egg in a small pot and cover it with water. Bring the water to a boil over high heat and boil for 12 minutes. Remove the egg, run it under cold water, peel away the shell, and cut in half.

3. In a bowl, whisk together the mayo, Parmesan, lemon juice, garlic, Worcestershire sauce, and Dijon mustard.

4. In a large bowl, combine the roasted red peppers, chickpeas, flax seeds, cherry tomatoes, shaved Parmesan, and kale. Top with the sliced chicken and hard-boiled egg, drizzle with the dressing, and serve.

Calories: 1,156 **Fat:** 55g **Carbs:** 79g **Fiber:** 22g **Sugar:** 12g **Protein:** 88g

Warm Harissa-Roasted Salmon Salad with Green Beans and Pistachios

I found this recipe for slow-roasted harissa salmon in an issue of *Bon Appétit* and fell in love, so I decided to build a salad around it. Harissa is a hot chili pepper paste that originated in North Africa but can be found at most grocery stores these days. The lemon, dill, and yogurt dressing offsets the spiciness of the harissa.

MAKES: 1 serving **TOTAL TIME:** 40 minutes

GF

1 lemon

2 tablespoons harissa paste

1 (8-ounce) skinless salmon fillet

¼ pound green beans, trimmed

¼ cup plain nonfat Greek yogurt

2 teaspoons lemon juice

½ teaspoon chopped fresh dill

3 cups mixed salad greens

½ cup cherry tomatoes, halved

¼ cup grated carrots

¼ cup shelled pistachios

1. Preheat the oven to 275°F. Cut three thin slices from the middle of the lemon and lay them in a small baking dish. Spread the harissa over the salmon and place it on top of the lemon slices. Roast until the salmon is cooked to your liking, about 30 minutes for medium-rare.

2. Bring 1 inch of water to a boil in a medium saucepan. Place the green beans in a steamer basket over the boiling water. Cover, turn the heat to medium, and steam for about 5 minutes, until they are bright green and just cooked.

3. In a small bowl, whisk together the yogurt, lemon juice, and dill.

4. Place the greens, tomatoes, carrots, and pistachios in a large bowl. Top with the salmon and green beans, drizzle with the dressing, and serve.

Calories: 1,208 **Fat:** 82g **Carbs:** 62g **Fiber:** 20g **Sugar:** 18g **Protein:** 85g

Shaved Brussels Sprouts Salad with Lentils and Kale

Most grocery stores carry pre-shredded Brussels sprouts if you're looking to save time. And feel free to replace the blue cheese with goat cheese if it's more to your liking or skip the cheese all together to make this salad plant-based. This recipe requires a few pots, but nothing is very hands on, so don't fear.

MAKES: 1 serving   **TOTAL TIME:** 50 minutes

GF

½ cup black beluga lentils

¼ cup quinoa

1 egg

2 cups Brussels sprouts, tough ends removed

2 cups baby arugula

1 cup shredded kale

3 tablespoons olive oil

1 large clove garlic, minced

1 tablespoon fresh lemon juice

¼ cup chopped walnuts

¼ cup dried cranberries

¼ cup crumbled blue cheese

salt

1. Fill a medium saucepan three quarters of the way with water. Add salt, then bring to a boil. Add the lentils, then turn the heat to medium-low and simmer for 25 minutes or until the lentils are tender but still firm. Drain well.

2. In a second saucepan, add the quinoa and ½ cup of water. Bring to a boil over high heat, then cover, turn the heat to low, and simmer for 15 minutes or until all the water has been absorbed.

3. Place the egg in a small pot and cover it with water. Bring the water to a boil over high heat and boil for 12 minutes. Remove the egg, run it under cold water, peel away the shell, and chop.

4. Using a knife, a mandolin slicer, or the slicing disk in your food processor, finely shred the Brussels sprouts. Place them in a bowl with the arugula and kale.

5. In a small bowl, whisk together the olive oil, garlic, lemon juice, and a pinch of salt and pepper. Pour half the dressing over the Brussels sprouts, arugula, and kale, and toss to coat.

6. Add the lentils, quinoa, egg, walnuts, cranberries, and blue cheese to the bowl. Drizzle with the remaining dressing and serve.

Calories: 1,136 **Fat:** 78g **Carbs:** 80g **Fiber:** 19g **Sugar:** 14g **Protein:** 42g

Chinese Steak Salad

Using the same mixture for the marinade and dressing makes for a tastier dish and cuts out a step in prep. Use coconut aminos instead of soy sauce to make this salad gluten-free.

MAKES: 1 serving   **TOTAL TIME:** 45 minutes

P

½ cup rice wine vinegar

1 tablespoon soy sauce

2 large cloves garlic, minced

1 teaspoon ground ginger

1 tablespoon brown sugar

1 teaspoon sesame oil

1 (6-ounce) sirloin steak

½ cup frozen shelled edamame beans

3 cups mixed salad greens

½ cup red cabbage

½ cup diced pineapple

¼ cup sliced almonds

½ cup grated carrots

1. In a bowl, combine the vinegar, soy sauce, garlic, ginger, brown sugar, and sesame oil. Reserve 3 tablespoons to use as dressing and pour the rest into a large zip-top bag with the steak. Seal and marinate in the fridge for at least 30 minutes.

2. Heat a grill or grill pan over medium heat. Remove the steak from the marinade and grill about 4 minutes per side for medium, or to desired doneness. Let it rest for 5 minutes then slice it into strips.

3. Cook the edamame beans according to the instructions on the package.

4. In a large bowl, combine the mixed greens, cabbage, pineapple, almonds, and carrots. Top with the edamame and sliced steak, drizzle with the dressing, and serve.

Calories: 827 Fat: 30g Carbs: 55g Fiber: 13g Sugar: 23g Protein: 70g

Quinoa and Kale Salad with Balsamic Vinaigrette

This salad is simple but loaded with filling fiber from the quinoa, squash, kale, and pumpkin seeds.

MAKES: 1 serving   **TOTAL TIME:** 30 minutes

GF, PB

½ cup red or tricolor quinoa

1 cup 1-inch pieces butternut squash

1 cup halved or quartered Brussels sprouts

salt, to taste

pepper, to taste

4 tablespoons olive oil, divided

1 tablespoon balsamic vinegar

1 teaspoon Dijon mustard

3 cups baby kale

2 tablespoons pumpkin seeds

¼ cup pecans, halved

1. Preheat the oven to 400°F. Cook the quinoa according to the package instructions.

2. Toss the butternut squash and Brussels sprouts with 1 table-spoon of olive oil and season with salt and pepper. Spread them in a single layer on a rimmed baking sheet and roast for 25 minutes.

3. In a small bowl, whisk together the remaining olive oil, balsamic vinegar, and Dijon mustard.

4. Place the kale in a large bowl. Top with the quinoa, squash, Brussels sprouts, pumpkin seeds, and pecans. Drizzle with the dressing and serve.

Calories: 1,154 **Fat:** 75g **Carbs:** 106g **Fiber:** 17g **Sugar:** 7g **Protein:** 27g

Kebab Salad with Pickled Onions

This falafel recipe makes 12 falafels, but you only need 4 for this salad. They keep well uncooked, so you can make the balls, just cook those you need, then refrigerate or freeze the rest. They also keep well cooked, so feel free to bake the whole batch. You'll find the same falafel in the Hummus and Falafel Bowl on page 128.

MAKES: 1 serving   **TOTAL TIME:** 1 hour

½ cup apple cider vinegar

4 teaspoons sugar

1 ½ teaspoons salt

½ red onion, thinly sliced

1 (15-ounce) can chickpeas, drained

4 large cloves garlic, peeled

2 shallots, peeled

2 tablespoons chopped fresh or 2 teaspoons dried parsley

1 teaspoon ground cumin

½ teaspoon ground coriander

½ teaspoon ground cardamom

3 tablespoons all-purpose flour

olive oil

¼ cup diced plus ½ cup grated and drained cucumber

½ cup plain Greek yogurt

1 teaspoon fresh lemon juice

2 teaspoons chopped fresh dill

2 teaspoons flax seeds

3 cups mixed salad greens

¼ cup banana peppers, sliced

¼ cup crumbled feta cheese

½ cup cherry tomatoes, halved

1. In a small bowl, combine the apple cider vinegar, sugar, and salt, and stir until the sugar and salt are dissolved. Add the red onion. Let it sit at room temperature for at least 1 hour.

2. In a food processor, combine the chickpeas, garlic, shallots, parsley, cumin, coriander, and cardamom. Pulse until the mixture resembles chunky hummus. Add the flour and pulse again to incorporate. Scoop some out and form a 2-inch ball or patty. If the mixture isn't holding together, add more flour 1 tablespoon at a time. Form 12 balls or disks. Place 4 on a baking sheet and freeze the rest.

3. Preheat the oven to 375°F. Brush the balls with a bit of olive oil or spray them with olive oil spray. Bake for 25 to 30 minutes, or until they are cooked through, rotating them halfway through cooking.

4. In a bowl, stir together the grated cucumber, yogurt, lemon juice, dill, and flax seeds.

5. Place the greens, banana peppers, feta, tomatoes, and diced cucumber in a large bowl. Top with the pickled onions and falafel, drizzle with the dressing, and serve.

Calories: 628 **Fat:** 17g **Carbs:** 88g **Fiber:** 18g **Sugar:** 21g **Protein:** 34g

Apple Walnut Chicken Salad with Creamy Sherry Vinaigrette

This is my spin on the Waldorf salad. The creamy sherry vinaigrette is inspired by the dressing on the Waldorf salad I used to order at Not Your Average Joe's when I was growing up.

MAKES: 1 serving   **TOTAL TIME:** 20 minutes

GF

1 (6-ounce) boneless, skinless chicken breast

¼ cup plain nonfat Greek yogurt

2 tablespoons sherry vinegar

1 tablespoon olive oil

½ teaspoon Dijon mustard

½ large or 1 small red apple, diced

⅓ cup raw walnut halves

¼ cup chopped dates

2 tablespoons crumbled goat cheese

¼ cup chopped celery

1 tablespoon flax seeds

3 cups romaine lettuce

salt and pepper

1. Heat a grill or grill pan over medium heat. Season the chicken with salt and pepper and grill until cooked through, 6 to 7 minutes per side, depending on thickness. Let it cool slightly then cut into strips.

2. In a bowl, whisk together the yogurt, sherry vinegar, olive oil, and Dijon mustard. Season with salt and pepper to taste.

3. In a large bowl, combine the apple, walnuts, dates, goat cheese, celery, flax seeds, and lettuce. Top with the chicken, drizzle with the dressing, and serve.

Calories: 832 Fat: 40g Carbs: 67g Fiber: 16g Sugar: 44g Protein: 55g

CHAPTER 8

One-Bowl Wonders

Fiery Mexican Burrito Bowl

I've been making a version of this recipe for years—it's super easy and delicious. Have fun with the toppings by subbing in guacamole for the avocado or throwing in some fresh or pickled jalapeños.

MAKES: 1 serving   **TOTAL TIME:** 45 minutes

GF

½ cup brown rice

2 tablespoon olive oil, divided

6 ounces lean ground beef

½ medium red, yellow, or orange bell pepper, stemmed, seeded, and sliced

¼ medium sweet onion, sliced

⅓ cup frozen corn

½ cup canned black beans, drained and rinsed

1 teaspoon chili powder

¼ teaspoon ground cumin

⅛ teaspoon paprika

⅛ teaspoon dried oregano

⅓ cup shredded Mexican cheese

¼ cup prepared salsa

½ avocado, peeled, pitted, and sliced

salt and pepper

1. Cook the rice according to the package instructions.

2. Heat 1 tablespoon of olive oil in a skillet over medium-high heat. Cook the ground beef in the oil, breaking it up with a wooden spoon until it is no longer pink, about 6 minutes. Season with salt and pepper and set aside.

3. Add the second tablespoon of oil, bell peppers, and onion to the skillet. Cook until soft, 5 to 6 minutes.

4. Return the ground beef to the skillet. Add the corn, black beans, chili powder, cumin, paprika, oregano, and a pinch of salt. Turn the heat to medium-low and stir until mixed and heated through, about 2 minutes.

5. Place the rice in a large bowl and top with the beef mixture, cheese, salsa, and avocado, and serve.

Calories: 1,464 Fat: 77g Carbs: 125g Fiber: 22g Sugar: 9g Protein: 78g

Fall Farro and Chicken Bowl with Roasted Vegetables

The hearty, chewy texture of farro is great for bowls. To better disperse the dressing, toss the farro with a bit of it before adding all the other components. I love all of these ingredients so much; this might be my favorite recipe in the whole book!

MAKES: 1 serving **TOTAL TIME:** 45 minutes

½ cup uncooked farro

1 (6-ounce) boneless, skinless chicken breast

1 cup Brussels sprouts, trimmed and halved or quartered, depending on size

½ cup 1-inch pieces butternut squash

2 tablespoons olive oil, divided

½ teaspoon salt, plus more for chicken

1 tablespoon plus ½ teaspoon pure maple syrup

2 teaspoons apple cider vinegar

2 teaspoons fresh lemon juice

¼ cup sliced cooked beets

2 tablespoons unsalted pumpkin seeds

⅛ cup crumbled goat cheese

¼ avocado, peeled, pitted, and sliced

½ cup baby arugula

pepper

1. Cook the farro according to the package instructions.

2. Preheat the oven to 400°F and grease a large rimmed baking sheet with cooking spray. Season the chicken with salt and pepper and place it on one side of the baking sheet. Toss the Brussels sprouts and butternut squash with 1 tablespoon of olive oil and the ½ teaspoon of salt, and spread them on the other side of the baking sheet. Roast for 30 minutes or until the chicken is cooked through. Chop the chicken into bite-size pieces.

3. While the chicken and veggies are roasting, whisk together the remaining olive oil, maple syrup, apple cider vinegar, lemon juice, and a pinch of salt and pepper.

4. Place the farro in a large bowl. Drizzle with 1 tablespoon of the dressing and mix. Top with the chicken, Brussels sprouts, butternut squash, beets, pumpkin seeds, goat cheese, avocado, and arugula. Drizzle with more of the dressing and serve.

Calories: 984 **Fat:** 51g **Carbs:** 80g **Fiber:** 16g **Sugar:** 20g **Protein:** 55g

Thai Peanut Noodle Bowl with Steak

The fresh, crunchy bean sprouts, cucumbers, and carrots mean that this bowl comes together really fast. I like to put the peanuts in a plastic bag, lay it on the counter, and use the bottom of a glass or a can to crush them.

MAKES: 1 serving   **TOTAL TIME:** 20 minutes

6 ounces whole wheat spaghetti

1 tablespoon olive oil

6 ounces steak tips or flank steak, sliced into strips

salt, to taste

pepper, to taste

⅛ cup creamy peanut butter

1 tablespoon rice or white vinegar

½ tablespoon soy sauce

1 teaspoon honey

pinch of ground ginger

1 ½ teaspoons water

1 cup bean sprouts

½ cucumber, seeds removed and sliced into 2-inch-long strips

1 carrot, shaved

2 tablespoons crushed peanuts

1. Cook the spaghetti according to the package instructions. Drain and place in a large bowl.

2. Heat the olive oil in a skillet over medium heat. Add the steak. Season with salt and pepper, and cook until just cooked through, about 6 minutes. Place in the bowl with the spaghetti.

3. In a bowl, combine the peanut butter, vinegar, soy sauce, honey, ginger, and water, and whisk until smooth. If the peanut butter is too difficult to whisk, blitz all the ingredients in a food processor until smooth.

4. Add the bean sprouts, cucumber, carrot, and peanut sauce to the bowl with the spaghetti and steak and toss to coat. Garnish with the crushed peanuts and serve.

Calories: 1,083 Fat: 55g **Carbs:** 80g **Fiber:** 13g **Sugar:** 17g **Protein:** 79g

Hummus and Falafel Bowl

Most people think of using a grain as the base for a bowl, but lentils are also a tasty and fiber-rich option. Omit the feta to make this one plant-based.

MAKES: 1 serving **TOTAL TIME:** 1 hour

½ cup apple cider vinegar

4 teaspoons sugar

1½ teaspoons salt

½ red onion, thinly sliced

1 (15-ounce) can chickpeas, drained

6 large cloves garlic, 4 peeled and 2 peeled and crushed

2 shallots, peeled

2 tablespoons chopped fresh or 2 teaspoons dried parsley

1 teaspoon ground cumin

½ teaspoon ground coriander

½ teaspoon ground cardamom

3 tablespoons all-purpose flour

¾ cup black beluga lentils

2 teaspoons olive oil

½ cucumber, diced

1 small tomato, seeds removed and diced

½ cup mixed greens

2 tablespoons crumbled feta cheese

2 tablespoons hummus

1 tablespoon tahini

½ lemon

1. In a small bowl, combine the apple cider vinegar, sugar, and salt, and stir until the sugar and salt are dissolved. Add the red onion. Let the onions sit at room temperature for at least 1 hour, until pickled.

2. In a food processor, combine the chickpeas, garlic, shallots, parsley, cumin, coriander, and cardamom. Pulse until the mixture resembles chunky hummus. Add the flour and pulse again to incorporate. Scoop some out and form a 2-inch ball or disk. If the mixture isn't holding together, add more flour 1 tablespoon at a time. Form 12 balls. Place 4 on a baking sheet and freeze the rest.

3. Preheat the oven to 375°F. Brush the balls with a bit of olive oil or spray them with olive oil spray. Bake for 25 to 30 minutes, or until they are cooked through, rotating them halfway through cooking.

4. Meanwhile, fill a medium saucepan three quarters of the way with water. Add salt, then bring to a boil. Add the lentils and crushed garlic, then turn the heat to medium-low and simmer for 25 minutes or until the lentils are tender but still firm. Drain well and toss with the olive oil.

5. Spoon the lentils into a bowl. Drain the pickled onions and add them to the bowl. Top with the falafel, cucumber, tomato, greens, feta, and hummus. Drizzle with the tahini and the juice from the lemon and serve.

Calories: 701 **Fat:** 27g **Carbs:** 92g **Fiber:** 21g **Sugar:** 16g **Protein:** 28g

Greek Quinoa Salmon Bowl

Cool, creamy tzatziki sauce, warm salmon, crunchy pistachios...this bowl is perfect no matter what you're craving.

MAKES: 1 serving   **TOTAL TIME:** 25 minutes

GF

½ cup quinoa

2 teaspoons olive oil

1 (8-ounce) salmon fillet

salt, to taste

½ cup plain nonfat Greek yogurt

½ cup grated cucumber, squeezed to drain

1 teaspoon fresh lemon juice

2 teaspoons chopped fresh dill

1 small clove garlic, minced

½ cup cherry tomatoes, halved

¼ cup diced red onion

¼ cup halved and pitted kalamata olives

¼ cup chopped fresh parsley

2 tablespoons crumbled feta cheese

2 tablespoons shelled pistachios

1. Cook the quinoa according to the package instructions.

2. Heat the olive oil in a skillet over medium-high heat. Pat the salmon dry with paper towels and season with salt.

3. Place the salmon in the pan and cook for 7 to 9 minutes, or until the light pink color is about ¾ of the way up the fillet. Flip and cook 2 minutes more, then transfer to a plate.

4. In a bowl, combine the Greek yogurt, grated cucumber, lemon juice, dill, and garlic, and stir to combine.

5. Spoon the quinoa into a bowl. Top with the cherry tomatoes, red onion, olives, parsley, feta, and pistachios. Lay the salmon fillet on top, drizzle with the tzatziki dressing, and serve.

Calories: 1,004 Fat: 46g Carbs: 78g Fiber: 12g Sugar: 10g Protein: 76g

Pesto Quinoa Bowl with Sundried Tomatoes

I've been making a pasta dish for a few years now with roasted asparagus, sundried tomatoes, mozzarella cheese, and pesto, and it's an amazing combination of flavors. So when I wanted to turn it into an OMAD meal, I kept all those flavors and upped the protein and fiber with quinoa, walnuts, and hard-boiled eggs.

MAKES: 1 serving   **TOTAL TIME:** 25 minutes

GF

½ cup quinoa

4 ounces asparagus, tough stems removed

2 teaspoons olive oil

sea salt, to taste

2 eggs

¼ cup basil pesto, divided

¼ cup peas, fresh or frozen and thawed

2 ounces fresh mozzarella, cubed

¼ cup sundried tomatoes, chopped

2 tablespoons chopped walnuts

1. Preheat the oven to 425°F. Cook the quinoa according to the package instructions.

2. Toss the asparagus with the olive oil and spread it in a single layer on a baking sheet. Sprinkle with sea salt and roast for 8 to 10 minutes.

3. Place the eggs in a small pot and cover them with water. Bring the water to a boil over high heat and boil for 12 minutes. Remove the eggs, run them under cold water, peel away the shells, and chop.

4. Spoon the quinoa into a bowl and stir in a tablespoon of the pesto. Top with the roasted asparagus, peas, mozzarella, sundried tomatoes, walnuts, and hard-boiled eggs. Spoon the remaining pesto over the top and serve.

Calories: 1,132 Fat: 69g Carbs: 80g Fiber: 14g Sugar: 14g Protein: 55g

Beet and Lentil Bowl with Creamy Lemon Dressing

If this recipe seems familiar as you're reading it, it's because this is the bowl on the cover of this book! Sliced jarred beets are a great option if you're short on time or, like me, are afraid of staining your entire kitchen when you peel the roasted beet.

MAKES: 1 serving **TOTAL TIME:** 1 hour

PB

1 whole raw beet, scrubbed, or 1 cup sliced jarred beets

½ cup black beluga lentils

½ cup broccoli florets

1 cup baby carrots with stems

2 ounces asparagus, tough stems removed and cut into 2-inch pieces

2 teaspoons fresh lemon juice

2 tablespoons olive oil

⅓ teaspoon Dijon mustard

½ teaspoon minced shallot

honey, to taste

½ cup canned chickpeas, drained and rinsed

3 radishes, quartered

½ avocado, peeled, pitted, and sliced

1. If you need to roast your beet, preheat the oven to 400°F. Wrap it loosely in tin foil, place it directly on the rack, and roast for about 50 minutes, or until you can easily pierce it with a fork. Let it cool slightly, then use a paper towel to rub off the skin. Cut it into chunks.

2. Fill a medium saucepan three quarters of the way with water. Add salt, then bring to a boil. Add the lentils, then turn the heat to medium-low and simmer for 25 minutes or until the lentils are tender but still firm. Drain well.

3. Bring 1 inch of water to a boil in a medium saucepan. Place the broccoli, carrots, and asparagus in a steamer basket over the boiling water. Cover, turn the heat to medium, and steam for about 5 minutes, until the veggies are brightly colored and just cooked.

4. In a small bowl, whisk together the lemon juice, olive oil, Dijon mustard, and minced shallot. Add a drop or two of honey to taste.

5. Place the beets, lentils, and steamed veggies in a large bowl. Top with the chickpeas, radishes, and avocado, drizzle everything with the dressing, and serve.

Calories: 787 **Fat:** 50g **Carbs:** 75g **Fiber:** 24g **Sugar:** 16g **Protein:** 19g

Beer-Breaded Fish Taco Rice Bowl

This bowl is inspired by my favorite dish from a restaurant aptly named Fish Taco. Because the fish does take some work, I wanted a super-simple dressing, so I had the idea to take some of the tangy juice from the jar of pickled jalapeños and stir it into some creamy Greek yogurt. Perfect!

MAKES: 1 serving   **TOTAL TIME:** 40 minutes

½ cup brown rice

¼ cup fresh or frozen and thawed corn

¼ cup diced tomatoes

2 teaspoons lime juice

¼ cup plus 2 tablespoons all-purpose flour

¼ teaspoon salt, plus more to taste

⅛ teaspoon pepper

¼ cup light Mexican beer, like Tecate or Modelo

¼ cup olive oil

1 (8-ounce) cod fillet, cut into strips

¼ cup pickled jalapeños

½ cup canned black beans, drained and rinsed

½ avocado, peeled, pitted, and sliced

¼ cup plain nonfat Greek yogurt

1 to 2 teaspoons pickled jalapeño juice from the jar

1. Cook the brown rice according to the package instructions.

2. In a bowl, combine the corn, diced tomatoes, and lime juice. Season with salt and put in the refrigerator until ready to eat.

3. In another bowl, mix the ¼ cup of flour, ¼ teaspoon of salt, pepper, and beer. Spread the remaining flour on a plate.

4. In a large high-sided skillet, heat the oil over medium heat until it sizzles when you drop a bit of batter in it.

5. Dip the fish strips into the flour, then the batter. Place them in the pan. Cook until golden brown and cooked through, about 2 to 3 minutes per side. Remove to a paper towel–lined plate.

6. Place the rice in a bowl. Top with the corn pico, jalapeños, black beans, avocado, and fish. Whisk together the Greek yogurt and jalapeño juice, drizzle it over everything, and serve.

Calories: 1,295 **Fat:** 40g **Carbs:** 156g **Fiber:** 22g **Sugar:** 9g **Protein:** 79g

Three Mushroom Sesame Black Rice Bowl

I love the meaty texture and umami flavor that mushrooms bring to a dish. Combine that with a dressing made with rice vinegar, ginger, soy sauce, and sesame oil and you've got a flavor explosion. Use coconut aminos in place of the soy sauce to make this gluten-free.

MAKES: 1 serving   **TOTAL TIME:** 45 minutes

PB

½ cup black or wild rice

3 tablespoons olive oil, divided

2 heads baby bok choy, leaves separated

2 carrots, peeled and sliced on the diagonal

½ cup sliced cremini mushrooms

¼ cup sliced shiitake mushrooms

½ cup sliced white mushrooms

1 large clove garlic, minced

salt, to taste

pepper, to taste

¼ cup halved cashews

¼ cup frozen shelled edamame beans

1 tablespoon rice vinegar

2 teaspoons soy sauce

1 teaspoon honey

⅛ teaspoon ground ginger

⅛ teaspoon sesame oil

¼ avocado, peeled, pitted, and sliced

1 tablespoon sesame seeds

1. Cook the rice according to the package instructions.

2. Heat 1 tablespoon of olive oil in a skillet over medium heat. Add the bok choy and carrots, and cook until starting to soften, about 4 minutes. Add the mushrooms and garlic, and season everything with salt and pepper. Cook until the mushrooms have released their liquid and the carrots and bok choy are tender, about 8 minutes more.

3. Spread the cashews on a small baking sheet or toaster oven tray. Heat the oven or toaster oven to 350°F. Add the cashews and toast (checking often, as these can burn very quickly) until the edges are just beginning to brown, about 3 minutes.

4. Cook the edamame according to the package instructions. In a bowl, whisk together the remaining 2 tablespoons of olive oil, rice vinegar, soy sauce, honey, ginger, and sesame oil. Add 1 tablespoon of the dressing to the rice and toss to coat.

5. Transfer the rice to a large bowl. Top with the mushroom mixture, edamame, cashews, and avocado. Drizzle with the remaining dressing, sprinkle with the sesame seeds, and serve.

Calories: 1,175 **Fat:** 78g **Carbs:** 101g **Fiber:** 16g **Sugar:** 17g **Protein:** 30g

Grain-less Bowl with Rosemary Potatoes and Turkey

I used to make a recipe similar to this all in a skillet, but it required a lot of stirring. So I decided to simplify it by roasting everything instead and then tossing in some crunchy pecans and apples for contrast. The result is autumn in a bowl!

MAKES: 1 serving   **TOTAL TIME:** 40 minutes

GF

8 ounces boneless, skinless turkey breast

2 teaspoons dried rosemary, divided

pinch of salt and pepper

3 to 4 mixed color baby potatoes, like purple, white, and sweet, cut into 1-inch pieces

1 cup halved Brussels sprouts

½ cup 1-inch pieces butternut squash

1 cup cauliflower florets

½ teaspoon ground cinnamon

½ teaspoon paprika

2 tablespoons olive oil

¼ cup diced cooked beets

¼ cup pecan halves

½ cup diced Granny Smith apples, peeled if desired

1. Preheat the oven to 400°F. Season the turkey with 1 teaspoon of rosemary and a pinch of salt and pepper. Place it on a large rimmed baking sheet.

2. Toss the potatoes, Brussels sprouts, butternut squash, and cauliflower with the remaining rosemary, cinnamon, paprika, and olive oil. Spread them on the baking sheet with the turkey.

3. Roast the turkey and veggies for about 30 minutes, until everything is tender. Cut the turkey into bite-size pieces.

4. Toss the turkey and roasted veggies in a bowl with the beets, pecans, and diced apples, and serve.

Calories: 1,038 Fat: 38g **Carbs:** 101g **Fiber:** 20g **Sugar:** 31g **Protein:** 99g

Sweet and Spicy Shrimp Soba Noodle Bowl

Soba noodles are thin, slightly nutty Japanese noodles made from gluten-free buckwheat flour. They're most often found in dishes with Asian flavor profiles, but you can use them in any of the noodle bowls in this chapter to make them gluten-free.

MAKES: 1 serving **TOTAL TIME:** 15 minutes

GF

6 ounces buckwheat soba noodles

4 ounces fresh or frozen and thawed shrimp, peeled, and deveined

salt, to taste

pepper, to taste

1 teaspoon Sriracha

2 tablespoons olive oil

1 tablespoon fresh lime juice

2 teaspoons honey

2 tablespoons apple cider vinegar

½ cup cherry tomatoes, halved

½ cup snow peas

¼ cup frozen and thawed corn

¼ cucumber, diced

½ avocado, peeled, pitted, and diced

4 green onions, sliced

1. Cook the soba noodles according to the package instructions.

2. Heat a grill or grill pan over medium heat. Season the shrimp with salt and pepper. Cook until the shrimp just turn pink, 1 to 2 minutes per side.

3. In a bowl, whisk together the Sriracha, olive oil, lime juice, honey, and apple cider vinegar.

4. In a large bowl, combine the shrimp, noodles, tomatoes, snow peas, corn, cucumber, avocado, and green onions. Toss with the dressing and serve.

Calories: 1,300 Fat: 52g Carbs: 172g Fiber: 12g Sugar: 19g Protein: 56g

Yellow Curry Bowl with Sweet Potato and Chickpeas

This recipe uses Thai yellow curry paste, a flavoring agent made from turmeric, curry powder, cumin, lemongrass, coriander, galangal, garlic, and dried chiles. You can find it online or in the international aisle at most grocery stores.

MAKES: 1 serving   **TOTAL TIME:** 40 minutes

PB

- ½ cup white or brown basmati rice, rinsed
- 2 teaspoons olive oil
- ¼ sweet onion, diced
- 2 carrots, peeled and diced
- 1 medium sweet potato, peeled, if desired, and diced
- ½ red bell pepper, cored and diced
- 3 tablespoons Thai yellow curry paste

- 1 teaspoon ground ginger
- 1 cup canned coconut milk
- ½ cup canned chickpeas, drained and rinsed
- 1 cup chopped kale, no ribs or stems
- 1 teaspoon brown sugar
- ½ teaspoon fish sauce or soy sauce
- ¼ cup chopped peanuts

1. Cook the basmati rice according to the package instructions.

2. Heat the olive oil in a skillet with a lid over medium heat. Add the onions and cook until soft, about 8 minutes.

3. Add the carrots, sweet potato, bell pepper, curry paste, ginger, and coconut milk, and stir to combine. Cover and cook, stirring occasionally, until the sweet potatoes are tender, about 12 minutes.

4. Stir in the chickpeas, kale, brown sugar, and fish sauce or soy sauce. Cook uncovered for another 5 minutes.

5. Place the rice in a bowl and spoon the curry on top. Garnish with the chopped peanuts and serve.

Calories: 1,257 **Fat:** 69g **Carbs:** 141g **Fiber:** 33g **Sugar:** 24g **Protein:** 30g

Loaded Beef Pad Thai

This takeout staple is surprisingly easy to make at home. Just make sure to have all your ingredients ready, as they cook fast.

MAKES: 1 serving   **TOTAL TIME:** 15 minutes

4 ounces brown rice noodles, like Annie Chun's

2 teaspoons olive oil

6 ounces sirloin steak, sliced into thin strips

salt, to taste

pepper, to taste

1 cup bean sprouts

4 green onions, sliced

½ red bell pepper, sliced into thin strips

2 heads baby bok choy, leaves separated

½ tablespoon soy sauce

1 tablespoon fish sauce

2 tablespoons brown sugar

1 tablespoon rice vinegar

½ teaspoon red pepper flakes

2 tablespoons chopped peanuts

1. Cook the noodles according to the package instructions. Drain and rinse with cold water.

2. Heat the olive oil in a large skillet over medium heat. Add the steak, season with salt and pepper, and cook for 6 minutes or until just cooked through. Remove and keep warm.

3. Add the bean sprouts, green onions, bell pepper, and bok choy to the skillet and cook until just soft, about 5 minutes.

4. In a small bowl, whisk together the soy sauce, fish sauce, brown sugar, rice vinegar, and red pepper flakes until the sugar is dissolved.

5. Add the noodles and steak to the skillet and pour in the sauce. Turn the heat to medium-low and toss until combined and heated through, about 2 minutes.

6. Serve garnished with the chopped peanuts.

Calories: 1,085 **Fat:** 32g **Carbs:** 128g **Fiber:** 15g **Sugar:** 28g **Protein:** 72g

Caribbean Shrimp Rice Bowl

This shrimp is flavored with jerk seasoning, which is a blend of chile peppers, salt, pepper, allspice, nutmeg, sugar, and thyme. Look for it in the spice aisle at your grocery store.

MAKES: 1 serving **TOTAL TIME:** 45 minutes

GF

½ cup brown rice

½ cup butternut squash, peeled and cut into 1-inch pieces

1 teaspoon olive oil

salt, to taste

pepper, to taste

4 ounces fresh or frozen and thawed shrimp, peeled and deveined

½ teaspoon jerk seasoning

¼ cup canned black beans, drained and rinsed

¼ cup diced fresh mango

¼ cup diced tomatoes

½ avocado, peeled, pitted, and diced

2 green onions, sliced

½ lime

1. Cook the brown rice according to the package instructions.

2. Preheat the oven to 375°F. Toss the butternut squash with the olive oil and season with salt and pepper. Spread the squash on a baking sheet and roast for 30 minutes.

3. Heat a grill or grill pan over medium heat. Toss the shrimp with the jerk seasoning. Cook until the shrimp just turn pink, 1 to 2 minutes per side.

4. Place the rice and butternut squash in a large bowl. Top with the shrimp, black beans, mango, tomatoes, avocado, and green onion. Drizzle with the juice of the lime and serve.

Calories: 864 **Fat:** 30g **Carbs:** 115g **Fiber:** 18g **Sugar:** 10g **Protein:** 41g

Farro and Salmon Bowl with Roasted Tomatoes and Pesto

The heat from the just-cooked farro is enough to wilt the spinach the perfect amount. Add in the soft and sweet roasted tomatoes and you've got a mouthwatering dish.

MAKES: 1 serving   **TOTAL TIME:** 20 minutes

K

- ½ cup farro
- 1 cup fresh baby spinach
- 2 teaspoons olive oil, divided
- 1 (8-ounce) salmon fillet
- 1 cup halved cherry or grape tomatoes
- salt, to taste
- pepper, to taste
- ½ cup canned cannellini beans, drained and rinsed
- 2 ounces mozzarella or burrata cheese
- ¼ cup basil pesto

1. Preheat the oven to 425°F. Cook the farro according to the package instructions. Strain out any liquid. Put the hot farro in a bowl, add the spinach, and cover the bowl so the spinach wilts.

2. Drizzle 1 teaspoon of olive oil over the salmon and toss the tomatoes with the other teaspoon. Season the salmon and tomatoes with salt and pepper. Place the salmon on a rimmed baking sheet and scatter the tomatoes around it. Roast for 12 minutes for salmon that's completely cooked through, or to your desired doneness.

3. Place the salmon and tomatoes in the bowl with the farro and spinach. Add the cannellini beans, cheese, and pesto, and serve.

Calories: 989 **Fat:** 60g **Carbs:** 40g **Fiber:** 10g **Sugar:** 9g **Protein:** 76g

Shrimp Teriyaki Stir-Fry

Stir fry is one of my go-to meals for days when I don't have much time to cook—I get the rice simmering while finishing other to-dos and the rest of the dish comes together in a flash. If you want to make this lighter, replace the basmati rice with cauliflower rice. You could also add some cauliflower rice to the basmati to bulk up the dish even more.

MAKES: 1 serving **TOTAL TIME:** 45 minutes

½ cup brown basmati rice, rinsed

1 tablespoon olive oil, divided

4 ounces fresh or frozen and thawed shrimp, peeled and deveined

salt, to taste

pepper, to taste

½ cup broccoli florets

4 ounces asparagus, chopped into bite-size pieces

¼ cup sliced mushrooms

½ red bell pepper, sliced

¼ cup baby corn

½ teaspoon ground ginger

¼ cup teriyaki sauce

¼ cup slivered almonds

1. Cook the rice according to the package instructions.

2. Heat 1 teaspoon of olive oil in a skillet over medium heat. Season the shrimp with salt and pepper, and cook until it just turns pink, 1 to 2 minutes per side. Set aside and keep warm.

3. Add the remaining oil to the skillet. Add the broccoli, asparagus, mushrooms, pepper, and baby corn, and cook until the broccoli is cooked through, about 7 minutes.

4. Return the shrimp to the pan. Add the ginger and teriyaki sauce, turn the heat to medium-low, and stir to combine. Cook until everything is warmed through, another minute or two.

5. Spoon the rice into a bowl. Top with the stir-fry mixture, garnish with the slivered almonds, and serve.

Calories: 819 **Fat:** 32g **Carbs:** 100g **Fiber:** 13g **Sugar:** 21g **Protein:** 45g

CHAPTER 9

Protein Plus Two

Steakhouse Classic with Garlic Herb Butter

It doesn't get any more classic than steak, asparagus, and a baked potato. Compound butters are an easy and delicious way to add flavor to meats.

MAKES: 1 serving **TOTAL TIME:** 1 hour

GF

- 1 clove garlic, minced
- 1 teaspoon finely chopped fresh parsley
- 1 teaspoon finely chopped fresh basil
- 2 tablespoons unsalted butter, softened
- 1 large russet potato
- 2 teaspoons olive oil, divided
- 8 ounces asparagus, tough stems removed
- 1 (7-ounce) sirloin steak
- salt and pepper

1. Preheat the oven to 350°F. In a small bowl, mix the garlic, parsley, and basil into the butter. Chill until ready to eat.

2. Prick the potato all over with a fork. Rub with 1 teaspoon of olive oil and season with salt and pepper. Place directly on the oven rack and roast until soft, about 60 minutes.

3. Heat a grill or grill pan over medium heat. Toss the asparagus with the remaining olive oil and season with salt. Season the steak with salt and pepper. Place both on the grill pan.

4. Grill the asparagus until you can pierce it easily with a fork, about 8 minutes. After 4 minutes, flip the steak and continue cooking for the remaining 4 minutes for medium, or to your desired doneness.

5. Serve the steak and asparagus alongside the baked potato and topped with the garlic herb butter.

Calories: 1,033 Fat: 51g Carbs: 74g Fiber: 12g Sugar: 8g Protein: 71g

Teriyaki Salmon with Orange Basmati Rice and Broccoli Rabe

The honey in the teriyaki glaze makes it thicken to sweet, syrupy goodness. Replace the soy sauce with coconut aminos to make it gluten-free.

MAKES: 1 serving   **TOTAL TIME:** 1 hour

4 tablespoons teriyaki sauce

¼ cup packed brown sugar

¾ teaspoon ground ginger

4 tablespoons soy sauce

1 tablespoon white vinegar

3 cloves garlic, minced

2 tablespoons honey

1 tablespoon sesame oil (optional)

1 (8-ounce) skin-on salmon fillet

½ cup orange juice

½ cup basmati rice, white or brown, rinsed

8 ounces broccoli rabe, tough stems removed

1 tablespoon olive oil

¼ cup slivered almonds

pinch of salt

1. Combine the teriyaki sauce, brown sugar, ginger, soy sauce, vinegar, garlic, honey, and sesame oil in a medium bowl. Place the salmon in the bowl, flesh-side down. Cover with plastic wrap and marinate for at least 20 minutes.

2. Meanwhile, bring ½ cup of water and the orange juice to a boil in a medium saucepan. Add the rice, turn the heat to low, cover, and simmer for 40 minutes or until all the water has been absorbed. Let it sit, covered, until ready to serve.

3. Preheat the oven to 400°F. Grease a rimmed baking sheet and place the salmon skin-side down on the baking sheet. Roast to your desired doneness, about 12 minutes for medium or 15 minutes for completely cooked through.

4. Bring 1 inch of water to a boil in a medium saucepan. Place the broccoli rabe in a steamer basket over the boiling water. Cover, turn the heat to medium, and steam for 5 minutes, or until the broccoli rabe is bright green and just cooked. Remove to a bowl and toss with the olive oil, slivered almonds, and a pinch of salt. Set aside until ready to serve.

5. While the salmon is cooking, pour the used marinade into a small saucepan. Bring it to a boil, then turn the heat to medium-low and simmer, uncovered, for 8 minutes or until thick and sticky.

6. To serve, place the salmon, rice, and broccoli rabe on a plate and drizzle everything with the teriyaki glaze.

Calories: 1,656 **Fat:** 59g **Carbs:** 208g **Fiber:** 29g **Sugar:** 96g **Protein:** 94g

Sheet Pan Chicken with Potatoes, Carrots, and Parsnips

I learned from my mom that if you're going to roast carrots, you should always roast parsnips alongside them. The key for even cooking is to make sure that the pieces of potato, carrot, and parsnip are all about the same size.

MAKES: 1 serving   **TOTAL TIME:** 35 minutes

GF

8 ounces boneless, skinless chicken breast or chicken thighs, pounded to uniform thickness

½ teaspoon garlic powder

1 teaspoon salt, divided

½ teaspoon pepper, divided

6 ounces baby red bliss or fingerling potatoes, quartered

2 carrots, peeled and sliced diagonally into 1-inch pieces

2 parsnips, peeled and sliced diagonally into 1-inch pieces

2 tablespoons olive oil

1 teaspoon dried rosemary

1½ teaspoons dried thyme

1. Preheat the oven to 400°F. Grease a large rimmed baking sheet or two small baking sheets with cooking spray. Season the chicken with the garlic powder, ½ teaspoon of salt, and ¼ teaspoon of pepper. Place on one side of the large baking sheet or one of the small ones.

2. In a bowl, toss the potatoes, carrots, and parsnips with the olive oil, rosemary, thyme, and remaining salt and pepper. Spread in a single layer on the other side of the baking sheet or on the second small one.

3. Roast everything for about 25 minutes or until the chicken is cooked through and the veggies are tender and starting to crisp around the edges. Serve.

Calories: 894 **Fat:** 35g **Carbs:** 93g **Fiber:** 22g **Sugar:** 21g **Protein:** 56g

Smothered Cheeseburger with Tater Tots

I started making this recipe one year during Passover and never stopped. Look for tater tots that only list potatoes on their ingredients list.

MAKES: 1 serving **TOTAL TIME:** 25 minutes

GF

10 ounces frozen tater tots

½ pound lean ground beef

1 to 2 teaspoons liquid smoke (optional)

salt, to taste

pepper, to taste

1 tablespoon olive oil

½ red or orange bell pepper, sliced

½ sweet onion, sliced

5 ounces sliced white mushrooms

1 ounce cheddar cheese, sliced

1. Cook the tater tots in the oven according to the package instructions.

2. Shape the ground beef into one large ball. Make a hole in the middle and pour in the liquid smoke, if using, then form into a patty. Season on both sides with salt and pepper, then use your thumb to press down and create a depression in the middle of the patty.

3. Heat the olive oil in a skillet over medium-high heat. Add the sliced bell pepper and onion and cook for 3 minutes. Add the sliced mushrooms and cook for 3 minutes more, or until all the veggies are soft.

4. Heat a griddle or grill pan over medium heat. Cook the burger for 4 minutes, then flip and cook 4 minutes more for medium.

Place the cheese on the burger and turn off the heat. Let the pan sit on the stove for another minute or so until the cheese is melted.

5. Put the cheeseburger on a plate and top it with the sautéed veggies. Serve immediately with the tater tots.

Calories: 1,376 **Fat:** 82g **Carbs:** 93g **Fiber:** 11g **Sugar:** 9g **Protein:** 71g

Balsamic Chicken and Broccoli with Cheddar Cauli-Potato Mash

You won't even notice the cauliflower in this mash, except for the fact that it doubles your portion size for a boost in satiety.

MAKES: 1 serving   **TOTAL TIME:** 1 hour 15 minutes

GF

8 ounces boneless, skinless chicken breasts or thighs

3 tablespoons olive oil, divided

¼ cup plus 2 tablespoons balsamic vinegar, divided

½ small head cauliflower, roughly chopped

1 medium russet potato, peeled and roughly chopped

1 small head or ½ large head broccoli, cut into florets

¼ cup heavy cream

¼ cup shredded cheddar cheese

¼ teaspoon salt, plus more to taste

pepper

1. Place the chicken in a large zip-top bag with 2 tablespoons of olive oil and ¼ cup of balsamic vinegar. Seal and let it marinate in the fridge for at least 30 minutes.

2. Preheat the oven to 400°F. Place the cauliflower and potato in a medium pot. Cover with water, add a pinch of salt, and bring to a boil. Once it's boiling, lower the heat to medium-low, cover, and simmer for 10 minutes, or until the cauliflower and potato are tender. Drain and return them to the pot.

3. Place the marinated chicken on half a large rimmed baking sheet or one small baking sheet. Toss the broccoli with the remaining olive oil and balsamic vinegar and place it on the other half of the large baking sheet or on its own small baking sheet.

Season the chicken and broccoli with salt and pepper. Roast for 25 minutes, or until the broccoli is tender and the chicken is cooked through.

4. Add the heavy cream, shredded cheddar, and salt to the pot with the potato and cauliflower, and use a potato masher to create a mash. If you prefer a smoother puree, place the cauliflower, potato, cream, cheddar, and salt in a food processor and blitz until smooth.

5. Serve the roasted chicken and broccoli alongside the cauliflower-potato mash.

Calories: 1,206 **Fat:** 70g **Carbs:** 62g **Fiber:** 12g **Sugar:** 20g **Protein:** 85g

Grilled Mahi Tacos with Cilantro Lime Rice and Avocado Crema

Mahi mahi is a light fish but it holds together quite well on the grill. Feel free to make the slaw ahead of time and let it sit in the fridge until serving.

MAKES: 1 serving   **TOTAL TIME:** 45 minutes

½ cup long grain white or brown rice

2 tablespoons fresh lime juice, divided

⅓ cup lightly packed chopped cilantro

1 teaspoon smoked paprika

⅛ teaspoon dried oregano

⅛ teaspoon dried thyme

½ teaspoon ground cumin

⅛ teaspoon chili powder

¼ teaspoon kosher salt, plus more to taste

1 (8-ounce) mahi mahi fillet

½ avocado, peeled and pitted

¼ cup plain nonfat Greek yogurt

½ cup diced fresh pineapple

½ cup red cabbage

¼ white onion, thinly sliced

¼ cup shredded carrots

⅛ cup pickled jalapeños

3 small corn tortillas, warmed

1. Cook the rice according to the package instructions. Remove from heat and stir in 1 tablespoon of lime juice and the cilantro. Cover to keep warm.

2. Heat a grill pan or a cast-iron skillet over medium-high and spray with cooking spray.

3. In a small bowl, mix together the smoked paprika, oregano, thyme, cumin, chili powder, and salt. Rub the mixture on both sides of the mahi mahi. Grill the fish 2 to 3 minutes per side.

4. In a food processor or blender, combine the avocado, Greek yogurt, ½ tablespoon of lime juice, and a pinch of salt. Blend until smooth.

5. In a bowl, toss the pineapple, cabbage, onion, carrots, jalapeños, the remaining ½ tablespoon of lime juice, and a pinch of salt.

6. Place the tortillas on a plate. Evenly divide the pineapple slaw among them. Break the fish up into pieces and divide it amongst the tacos. Top with the avocado crema and serve alongside the cilantro lime rice.

Calories: 1,052 **Fat:** 27g **Carbs:** 142g **Fiber:** 21g **Sugar:** 18g **Protein:** 65g

Orange Juice Chicken with Crispy Cauliflower and Quinoa

This chicken is sweet, tangy, and full of flavor. To avoid covering your kitchen with tiny pieces of cauliflower, use kitchen shears to turn the head into florets.

MAKES: 1 serving   **TOTAL TIME:** 45 minutes

1⅓ tablespoons unsalted butter

8 ounces boneless, skinless chicken breast

⅓ teaspoon salt

2 teaspoons all-purpose flour

1 teaspoon sugar

pinch of dry mustard

pinch of ground cinnamon

pinch of ground ginger

½ cup orange juice

½ head cauliflower, cut into florets

2 tablespoons olive oil

½ teaspoon dried thyme

½ cup quinoa

½ cup chicken broth

1. Preheat the oven to 425°F. Melt the butter in a skillet with a lid over medium heat. Brown the chicken on both sides, about 3 minutes per side, then remove from the skillet.

2. Add the salt, flour, sugar, dry mustard, cinnamon, and ginger to the skillet. Stir the mixture until it forms a smooth paste. Slowly stir in the orange juice and bring to a boil.

3. While you're waiting for the sauce to boil, toss the cauliflower florets in a bowl with the olive oil and thyme. Spread on a rimmed baking sheet and roast until tender and crisp, about 20 minutes.

4. Return the chicken to the skillet. Cover, reduce the heat to low, and cook until the chicken is tender, about 20 minutes.

5. Meanwhile, place the quinoa, chicken broth, and ½ cup of water in a medium pot. Bring to a boil, cover, and simmer for 15 minutes, until all the liquid has been absorbed.

6. Serve the chicken alongside the cauliflower and quinoa, all drizzled with the orange juice sauce.

Calories: 1,069 **Fat:** 54g **Carbs:** 83g **Fiber:** 10g **Sugar:** 18g **Protein:** 64g

Loaded BBQ Baked Potato

If you're not in a chicken mood, you could also make this dish with the barbecue pulled pork in Chapter 11, page 224.

MAKES: 1 serving   **TOTAL TIME:** 1 hour 30 minutes

GF

½ cup ketchup

2 tablespoons brown sugar

2 teaspoons apple cider vinegar

2 teaspoons Worcestershire sauce

1 teaspoon smoked paprika

¼ teaspoon salt, plus more to taste

pepper, to taste

1 (6-ounce) boneless, skinless chicken breast or thigh, cut into a few pieces

1 large russet potato

1 teaspoon olive oil

2 slices bacon

2 green onions, chopped

¼ cup shredded cheddar cheese

½ avocado, peeled, pitted, and diced

sour cream (optional)

1. In a bowl, stir together the ketchup, brown sugar, apple cider vinegar, Worcestershire sauce, smoked paprika, salt, and pepper. Pour it into a large zip-top bag. Add the chicken and marinate for at least 20 minutes.

2. Preheat the oven to 350°F. Prick the potato all over with a fork. Rub with 1 teaspoon of olive oil and season with salt and pepper. Place directly on the oven rack and roast until soft, about 60 minutes.

3. Place the chicken in a baking dish. When the potato has 30 minutes to go, put the chicken in the oven to roast alongside it for the last 30 minutes.

4. While the chicken and potato are cooking, place the bacon on a paper towel–lined plate. Microwave on high for 5 minutes, or until crispy. Let it cool slightly before chopping.

5. Pour the barbecue marinade into a small pot. Bring to a boil over high heat and boil for 2 minutes.

6. Shred the chicken and toss it in the pot with the barbecue sauce.

7. Cut the potato open horizontally. Top it with the chicken, bacon, green onions, shredded cheese, avocado, and sour cream, if desired, and serve.

Calories: 1,318 **Fat:** 56g **Carbs:** 127g **Fiber:** 17g **Sugar:** 51g **Protein:** 83g

Steak and Shrimp with Garlic Mashed Potatoes and Grilled Zucchini

This take on restaurant surf and turf is simple, yet decadent. Be sure not to slice the zucchini so thin that it falls apart on the grill.

MAKES: 1 serving   **TOTAL TIME:** 30 minutes

GF

2 large or 3 small red bliss potatoes

1 large clove garlic

½ tablespoon unsalted butter

2 tablespoons heavy cream

1 medium zucchini

1 teaspoon olive oil

1 teaspoon Italian seasoning

½ teaspoon dried thyme

1 (5-ounce) sirloin steak

3 fresh or frozen and thawed jumbo shrimp

salt, to taste

pepper, to taste

1. Place the potatoes and garlic in a medium pot. Cover with water and bring to a boil over high heat. Cover, turn the heat to medium-low, and simmer until the potatoes are tender, about 15 minutes. Drain well and return the potatoes and garlic to the pot. Add the butter and cream and use a potato masher to mash. Cover to keep warm, if needed.

2. Slice the ends off the zucchini then cut it in half crosswise (so you now have two smaller zucchini). Cut each half lengthwise into ¾-inch-thick planks. Toss the zucchini planks with the olive oil, Italian seasoning, and thyme.

3. Heat a grill or grill pan over medium heat. Season the steak and shrimp with salt and pepper. Place the steak, shrimp, and zucchini on the grill. After 2 minutes, flip the shrimp and the zucchini. After 4 minutes, remove the shrimp and the zucchini, and flip the steak. Continue cooking the steak to your desired doneness, about 4 minutes more for medium.

4. Serve the steak, shrimp, and zucchini with the garlic mashed potatoes.

Calories: 936 **Fat:** 33g **Carbs:** 79g **Fiber:** 10g **Sugar:** 11g **Protein:** 85g

Rosemary-Garlic Pork Chops with Lentil Pilaf

Creating a pilaf with lentils instead of rice adds a hearty helping of fiber to this meal.

MAKES: 1 serving **TOTAL TIME:** 40 minutes

GF

½ cup chicken broth

½ cup black beluga lentils

2 large cloves garlic, minced and divided

1 (6-ounce) bone-in pork loin chop

1 teaspoon olive oil

2 tablespoons unsalted butter, melted

1 teaspoon dried rosemary

½ cup 1-inch pieces butternut squash

2 tablespoons chopped pecans

2 tablespoons dried cranberries

salt and pepper

1. Pour the chicken broth into a medium saucepan, then fill it with water until it is three-quarters of the way full. Add a pinch of salt, then bring to a boil. Add the lentils and 1 minced clove garlic, then turn the heat to medium-low and simmer for 25 minutes or until the lentils are tender but still firm. Drain well.

2. Preheat the oven to 375°F. Season the pork chop with salt and pepper. Heat the olive oil in an oven-safe skillet over medium-high heat. Sear the pork chop until golden on both sides, 3 to 4 minutes per side.

3. In a small bowl, mix the remaining garlic with the butter and rosemary. Brush the butter mixture on both sides of the pork chop.

4. Transfer the skillet to the oven and cook until the chop is cooked through, about 10 minutes more.

5. While the pork is in the oven, place the butternut squash in a microwave-safe dish. Cover and microwave on high until tender, about 10 minutes.

6. Spread the chopped pecans on a small baking sheet or toaster oven tray. If you're using a toaster oven, heat it to 350°F and toast the pecans until the edges are just beginning to brown, about 3 minutes. If you're using the oven, put them in when the pork has 3 minutes left.

7. Toss the lentils with the squash, cranberries, pecans, and a drizzle of olive oil. Serve alongside the pork chop.

Calories: 938 **Fat:** 45g **Carbs:** 76g **Fiber:** 33g **Sugar:** 6g **Protein:** 59g

Giant Italian Meatball Stacker

Regardless of whether you call this a giant meatball or an Italian burger, it is deliciously juicy. For additional flair and flavor, drizzle a bit of balsamic vinegar over the stack before eating.

MAKES: 1 serving   **TOTAL TIME:** 15 minutes

K

½ pound Italian sausage or ground beef

2 tablespoons basil pesto

2 tablespoons panko breadcrumbs

2 tablespoons grated Parmesan cheese

2 tablespoons milk

2 (1-inch-thick) slices eggplant

1 portobello mushroom cap

2 teaspoons olive oil

salt, to taste

pepper, to taste

1 teaspoon Italian seasoning

2 (1-inch-thick) slices tomato

2 ounces mozzarella cheese

¼ cup fresh basil leaves, shredded

1. In a bowl, combine the sausage or ground beef, pesto, breadcrumbs, Parmesan, and milk, and form into a patty.

2. Heat a grill or grill pan over medium heat. Drizzle the eggplant and portobello mushroom with the olive oil and season with the Italian seasoning, salt, and pepper.

3. Grill the patty, eggplant slices, and portobello mushroom cap about 4 minutes per side or until the patty is cooked to your liking.

4. Place one of the eggplant slices on your plate. Top with a tomato slice, then the patty, then the mozzarella, then the mushroom cap. Finish with the second tomato slice and second eggplant slice. Sprinkle with the fresh basil and serve.

Calories: 1,061 **Fat:** 80g **Carbs:** 30g **Fiber:** 5g **Sugar:** 11g **Protein:** 58g

California Turkey Burger with Sweet Potato Fries

What happens when you combine two delicious condiments in Sriracha and ranch dressing? You get a super condiment that gives this burger just enough of a kick. Feel free to melt a slice of cheddar or pepper jack cheese on top too, if you'd like.

MAKES: 1 serving   **TOTAL TIME:** 30 minutes

½ pound 94% lean ground turkey

1 ½ tablespoons whole wheat breadcrumbs

1 small clove garlic, minced

1 teaspoon Worcestershire sauce

1 tablespoon chopped fresh parsley or cilantro

1 large sweet potato, peeled if desired and cut into 1-inch-wide wedges

1 tablespoon olive oil

1 teaspoon chili powder

½ teaspoon kosher salt

2 teaspoons ranch dressing

½ teaspoon Sriracha

1 whole wheat hamburger bun

½ cup fresh baby spinach

3 slices red onion

¼ avocado, peeled, pitted, and sliced

1. In a bowl, combine the ground turkey, breadcrumbs, garlic, Worcestershire sauce, and chopped parsley or cilantro. Shape into a patty and chill while you prepare the fries.

2. Preheat the oven to 450°F. In a bowl, toss the sweet potato wedges with the olive oil, chili powder, and kosher salt. Spread them in a single layer in a large glass baking dish or on a heavy rimmed baking sheet. Roast for 20 minutes, turning halfway through.

3. Heat a grill, grill pan, or griddle pan to medium heat. Spray it with cooking spray and cook the turkey burger for 5 minutes, then flip and cook 5 minutes more, or until the center is no longer pink.

4. Mix together the ranch dressing and Sriracha and spread it on the bottom bun. Top with the burger, spinach, onion, avocado, and top bun. Serve with the sweet potato fries.

Calories: 1,022 **Fat:** 56g **Carbs:** 71g **Fiber:** 15g **Sugar:** 19g **Protein:** 72g

Old Bay Salmon with Roasted Veggie Quinoa Salad

This is my homage to my current home state of Maryland and its pride and joy, Old Bay seasoning, which always reminds me of summer. The fresh quinoa salad is the perfect accompaniment for the flavor-packed salmon.

MAKES: 1 serving   **TOTAL TIME:** 25 minutes

GF

½ cup tricolored quinoa

1 (8-ounce) salmon fillet

1 tablespoon olive oil, divided

2 teaspoons Old Bay seasoning

½ summer squash, diced

½ cup cherry tomatoes, halved

½ cup diced red onion

salt, to taste

pepper, to taste

¼ cup slivered almonds

1 lemon, halved

1. Preheat the oven to 425°F. Cook the quinoa according to the package instructions.

2. Rub the salmon on all sides with 1 teaspoon of olive oil and the Old Bay seasoning, and place it on a large baking sheet. Toss the squash, tomatoes, and onion with another teaspoon of olive oil, season with salt and pepper, and spread in a single layer on the baking sheet.

3. Roast the salmon and veggies until the salmon is cooked to your liking, about 15 minutes for cooked through.

4. In a bowl, toss the quinoa with the veggies, almonds, remaining teaspoon of olive oil, and the juice from half the lemon.

5. Drizzle the salmon with the juice from the other half of the lemon and serve alongside the quinoa salad.

Calories: 935 Fat: 46g Carbs: 76g Fiber: 14g Sugar: 9g Protein: 64g

Honey-Glazed Pork Chop with Acorn Squash and Kale

The skin of acorn squash gets soft and tender when roasted, so there's no need to peel it, making this dish super simple to make.

MAKES: 1 serving   **TOTAL TIME:** 25 minutes

P, GF

3 tablespoons raw honey

1 ½ tablespoons finely chopped fresh sage or 1 ¼ teaspoons dried sage

2 large cloves garlic, minced

1 (6-ounce) boneless pork loin chop

salt, to taste

pepper, to taste

½ medium acorn squash, ends removed, seeded, and sliced

2 cups curly kale, ribs and stems removed

1. Preheat the oven to 400°F. Microwave the honey for 15 seconds, then whisk in the sage and garlic. Season the pork chop on both sides with salt and pepper.

2. Brush 1 tablespoon of the honey mixture over the pork chop. Toss the acorn squash and kale with a second tablespoon of the honey mixture. Reserve the final tablespoon.

3. Place the pork on a rimmed baking sheet. Spread the squash slices and kale around it. Roast for about 20 minutes, flipping the pork chop halfway through, or until the pork is cooked to your desired doneness.

4. Microwave the final tablespoon of sage honey for 15 seconds or until liquefied. Drizzle it over everything and serve.

Calories: 819 Fat: 13g Carbs: 124g Fiber: 13g Sugar: 52g Protein: 63g

CHAPTER 10

Steaming Chilis and Soups

Sweet and Spicy Turkey Chili

This is my mom's go-to chili recipe. You can simmer it in a pot on the stove, which is the way the recipe is written here. Or if you'd prefer, you can complete step 1 using a skillet then transfer all the ingredients (minus the shredded cheese) to a slow cooker and let the chili come together on low for 4 to 6 hours. Either way, you'll have a tasty and heartwarming chili come mealtime!

MAKES: 6 servings   **TOTAL TIME:** 1 hour

GF

2 tablespoons olive oil, divided

1 white or sweet onion, chopped

2 bell peppers, any color, cored and chopped

1½ pounds ground turkey

1 (28-ounce) can stewed tomatoes

1 (6-ounce) can tomato paste

1 (12-ounce) bottle chili sauce, like Heinz

1 cup red wine

1 tablespoon brown sugar

1 tablespoon chili powder

1 (15-ounce) can dark red kidney beans, drained and rinsed

1 (15-ounce) can red kidney beans, drained and rinsed

1 (14.5-ounce) can chickpeas, drained and rinsed

1 cup shredded cheddar cheese

1. In a stockpot or Dutch oven, heat 1 tablespoon of olive oil over medium heat. Add the onion and peppers and cook until they start to soften, 5 to 6 minutes. Add the ground turkey and cook, breaking it up with a wooden spoon until browned, about 10 minutes.

2. Add all the remaining ingredients except the shredded cheese to the pot and stir to combine. Turn the heat to high, bring it to a boil, then turn to medium-low and simmer at least 30 minutes to allow the flavors to come together.

3. Serve in bowls topped with the shredded cheese.

Calories: 661 **Fat:** 26g **Carbs:** 59g **Fiber:** 15g **Sugar:** 15g **Protein:** 51g

---

Fast Green Chicken Chili

I stole the idea of using jarred salsa to flavor chili from a recipe I found in *Cook's Country* magazine. It's a super-simple way to develop strong flavors as well as control the amount of heat in the dish. You could sub in red salsa for the green if you'd prefer. And if you're short on time, skip step 1 and instead pick up a rotisserie chicken, pull off the meat, and stir it into the chili during the last 5 minutes of cooking.

MAKES: 4 servings   **TOTAL TIME:** 45 minutes

K, GF

1 pound boneless, skinless chicken breasts and thighs

2 tablespoons olive oil, divided

salt, to taste

pepper, to taste

1 white onion, chopped

2 small cloves garlic, minced

2 teaspoons ground cumin

4 cups chicken broth

1 (15-ounce) can cannellini beans, drained and rinsed

1 (15-ounce) can black beans, drained and rinsed

1 cup jarred green salsa

¼ to ½ cup pickled jalapeños, depending on spice preference

1 cup crumbled cotija cheese

2 avocados, peeled, pitted, and diced

1. Preheat the oven to 375°F. Drizzle the chicken with 1 tablespoon of olive oil and season with salt and pepper. Roast about 30 minutes, or until cooked through. Use two forks to shred it into bite-size pieces.

2. Add the remaining oil to a Dutch oven or stockpot over medium heat. Add the onion and cook until beginning to soften, about 4 minutes. Stir in the garlic and cumin.

3. Add the broth, beans, salsa, and jalapeños to the pot. Turn the heat to high and bring to a boil, then reduce the heat to medium-low and simmer for 15 minutes, adding the shredded chicken for the last 5 minutes.

4. Serve the chili in bowls topped with cotija cheese and diced avocado.

Calories: 804 **Fat:** 41g **Carbs:** 51g **Fiber:** 21g **Sugar:** 7g **Protein:** 61g

Two-Bean Beef Chili with Sweet Potatoes

Growing up, we always had chili made with ground meat or ground turkey. Then I got my favorite cookbook, America's Test Kitchen's *One-Pan Wonders*, a few years ago and fell in love with a chili recipe made with beef chuck roast. If your grocery store doesn't sell chuck roast but does have packages of beef stew meat, that's actually even easier to use—and just as delicious.

MAKES: 6 servings   **TOTAL TIME:** 1 hour 45 minutes

GF

2 tablespoons olive oil, divided

3 pounds boneless beef chuck roast or stew meat, cut into 1-inch pieces

1 white or sweet onion, chopped

1 bell pepper, chopped

3 carrots, peeled and chopped

2 sweet potatoes, peeled or unpeeled (depending on your preference) and cut into ½-inch pieces

3 cloves garlic, minced

1 tablespoon chili powder

1 tablespoon ground cumin

1 tablespoon dried oregano

1 (28-ounce) can diced tomatoes and their juices

1 (15-ounce) can black beans, drained and rinsed

1 (15-ounce) can red kidney beans, drained and rinsed

1 (15-ounce) can chickpeas, drained and rinsed

1½ cups beer or beef broth

1½ cups shredded cheddar cheese

1. Preheat the oven to 350°F. Heat 1 tablespoon of olive oil in a Dutch oven over medium heat. Add half the beef and brown it on all sides, 6 to 8 minutes. Use tongs to transfer the beef to a bowl, and repeat with the remaining beef.

2. Add the second tablespoon of oil to the pot. Add the onion, bell pepper, carrots, and sweet potatoes, and cook until starting to soften, 5 to 6 minutes.

3. Add the garlic, chili powder, cumin, and oregano, and cook 1 minute. Add the diced tomatoes, beans, chickpeas, beer or broth, and browned beef and bring to a simmer.

4. Cover the pot and transfer it to the oven. Cook until beef is tender, 1 hour to 1 hour and 15 minutes.

5. Serve the chili topped with shredded cheese.

Calories: 949 **Fat:** 31g **Carbs:** 73g **Fiber:** 18g **Sugar:** 9g **Protein:** 91g

Chunky Minestrone Soup

Don't forget the grated Parmesan—it's what takes this veggie-packed soup to the next level. But if you want to make your meal plant-based, you can skip it.

MAKES: 4 servings   **TOTAL TIME:** 30 minutes

2 teaspoons olive oil

1 large white onion, chopped

4 carrots, peeled, halved lengthwise, and sliced

3 large cloves garlic, minced

1 (28-ounce) can diced tomatoes

3¾ cups vegetable broth

1 teaspoon Italian seasoning

1 teaspoon dried basil

1½ cups whole wheat pasta, like shells or elbows

1 medium zucchini, halved lengthwise and sliced

1 (15-ounce) can cannellini beans, drained and rinsed

1 cup fresh or frozen spinach

1 teaspoon Sriracha

salt, to taste

pepper, to taste

½ cup grated Parmesan cheese

1. In a large stockpot or Dutch oven, heat the oil over medium-high heat. Add the onion, carrots, and garlic, and cook for 3 minutes, until just starting to soften.

2. Add the tomatoes and their juices, broth, Italian seasoning, and basil. Turn the heat to high and bring to a boil, then cover, reduce the heat to medium-low, and simmer for 10 minutes.

3. Add the pasta, cover, and simmer for 10 minutes, stirring occasionally.

4. Add the zucchini, beans, spinach, and Sriracha, and simmer for 5 minutes more. Season to taste with salt and pepper and serve topped with grated Parmesan.

Calories: 658 Fat: 8g Carbs: 114g Fiber: 34g Sugar: 14g Protein: 41g

Mushroom and Barley Soup

I went to college in the middle of Connecticut, but 25 minutes from my school was the most incredible Jewish deli with the most incredible mushroom barley soup. It was savory, steamy, and so filling. I added some mild white beans to my version for additional protein and fiber.

MAKES: 4 servings   **TOTAL TIME:** 1 hour

PB

2 quarts beef or vegetable broth

2 bay leaves

2 large cloves garlic, crushed

1½ cups barley

1 tablespoon olive oil

1 white onion, chopped

6 carrots, peeled and chopped

4 celery stalks, chopped

1½ pounds mixed mushrooms

2 teaspoons dried thyme

1 cup canned cannellini beans, drained and rinsed

1. Pour the beef or vegetable broth into a large stockpot or Dutch oven and bring it to a boil over high heat. Once it's boiling, add the bay leaves, garlic and barley, then turn the heat to medium-low and let it simmer while you do the next step.

2. In a large skillet, heat the olive oil over medium heat. Add the onion, carrots, and celery, and cook until starting to soften, about 8 minutes. Add the mushrooms and thyme, and cook about 5 minutes more, until everything has started to brown.

3. Transfer the veggies to the stockpot. Stir in the cannellini beans and let everything simmer for another 20 to 30 minutes. Remove the bay leaves and serve.

Calories: 483 Fat: 8g Carbs: 79g Fiber: 20g Sugar: 12g Protein: 27g

Savory Lentil and Sausage Soup

Italian sausage soup and lentil soup are both delicious on their own, so why not combine them to make a hearty meal that's loaded with fiber? That was my thinking, at least.

MAKES: 4 servings   **TOTAL TIME:** 45 minutes

GF

2 teaspoons olive oil

1 pound Italian sausage, casings removed

1 large onion, chopped

4 carrots, peeled and chopped

2 celery stalks, chopped

1 (14.5-ounce) can crushed tomatoes

2 quarts beef broth

1 cup dry red lentils

1 (15-ounce) can kidney beans, drained and rinsed

1 teaspoon dried basil

1 teaspoon dried oregano

2 bay leaves

1 cup fresh or frozen spinach

1. In a large stockpot or Dutch oven, heat the olive oil over medium heat. Add the Italian sausage and cook, breaking it up with a wooden spoon, for 4 minutes. Add the onion, carrots, and celery, and continue to cook for 5 minutes.

2. Add the tomatoes, broth, lentils, beans, basil, oregano, and bay leaves. Turn the heat to high to bring it to a boil, then turn the heat to medium-low and simmer until the lentils are tender, at least 30 minutes.

3. Stir in the spinach and simmer for 5 minutes more. Remove the bay leaves and serve.

Calories: 831 **Fat:** 38g **Carbs:** 67g **Fiber:** 27g **Sugar:** 15g **Protein:** 54g

Turkey Tortilla Soup

To make this soup even faster, cook the turkey separately, shred it, and add it to the soup at step 4. You could also use a rotisserie chicken. It's garnished with avocado and shredded cheddar, but feel free to sprinkle on some crushed tortilla chips too.

MAKES: 4 servings **TOTAL TIME:** 50 minutes

K, GF

2 teaspoons olive oil

1 white onion, diced

2 jalapeños, diced

1 cup frozen corn

1 (15-ounce) can black beans, drained and rinsed

1 (14.5-ounce) can fire-roasted or crushed tomatoes

2 quarts chicken broth

1 tablespoon chipotle in adobo, minced (optional)

1 tablespoon paprika

2 teaspoons ground cumin

1 teaspoon chili powder

1 pound boneless, skinless turkey breast

2 tablespoons lime juice

½ cup roughly chopped cilantro leaves

1 avocado, peeled, pitted, and diced

1 cup shredded cheddar cheese

1. In a large stockpot or Dutch oven, heat the olive oil over medium heat. Add the onion and jalapeños, and cook for 5 minutes to soften.

2. Add the corn, black beans, tomatoes, chicken broth, chipotle, paprika, cumin, and chili powder. Turn the heat to high and bring it to a boil. Turn the heat to medium-low and simmer for 10 minutes.

3. Add the turkey and simmer until it is cooked through, 20 to 25 minutes.

4. Remove the turkey, shred it with two forks, then return it to the pot along with the lime juice and cilantro. Serve the soup garnished with avocado and shredded cheese.

Calories: 648 **Fat:** 27g **Carbs:** 46g **Fiber:** 17g **Sugar:** 11g **Protein:** 57g

Creamy Chicken and Wild Rice Soup

This soup is lower in fiber than some of the others in this chapter, but its thick, creamy base makes it feel hearty, indulgent, and satisfying as you eat it. The smaller you cut the chicken the faster it will cook, but feel free to let it simmer for as long as you need—because it's cooking in the broth, it will stay nice and juicy and delicious.

MAKES: 4 servings   **TOTAL TIME:** 1 hour

2 teaspoons olive oil

4 carrots, peeled and sliced

1 white onion, chopped

1 green bell pepper, chopped

1 cup sliced mushrooms

3 large cloves garlic, minced

1 teaspoon dried thyme

1 teaspoon dried oregano

¼ cup all-purpose flour

1 cup wild rice

½ cup black beluga lentils

2 quarts chicken broth

2 cups water

1 pound boneless skinless chicken breast, cut into bite-size pieces

1 cup heavy cream

salt and pepper

1. In a large stockpot or Dutch oven, heat the olive oil over medium heat. Add the carrots, onion, bell pepper, and mushrooms, and cook for 5 minutes to soften. Add the garlic, thyme, and oregano, and cook for 1 minute more. Sprinkle the flour over the vegetables and cook, stirring, for 3 minutes.

2. Add the rice, lentils, chicken broth, and water. Turn the heat to high and bring the mixture to a boil, then turn to medium-low and simmer for 20 minutes.

3. Add the chicken and simmer for 20 minutes more, or until it is cooked through and the rice and lentils are tender.

4. Stir in the cream, season with salt and pepper to taste, and serve.

Calories: 733 **Fat:** 26g **Carbs:** 67g **Fiber:** 13g **Sugar:** 9g **Protein:** 58g

Italian Sausage and Tortellini Soup

What's better than noodles in soup? Cheese in noodles in soup! The tortellini and diced potatoes give this thick soup a stew-like quality that makes it extra heartwarming and filling.

MAKES: 4 servings   **TOTAL TIME:** 55 minutes

1 tablespoon olive oil

1 pound Italian sausage, casings removed

1 white onion, chopped

3 large cloves garlic, minced

1 (28-ounce) can diced or crushed tomatoes

2 russet or Yukon gold potatoes, diced

1 cup cannellini beans, drained and rinsed

1 (8-ounce) can tomato sauce

2 quarts beef broth

½ cup red wine

1 teaspoon dried basil

1 teaspoon dried oregano

1 medium zucchini, halved lengthwise and sliced

8 ounces cheese tortellini

2 cups fresh baby spinach

½ cup grated Parmesan cheese

1. In a large stockpot or Dutch oven, heat the oil over medium heat. Add the sausage and cook, breaking it up into smaller pieces with a wooden spoon, about 10 minutes. Remove to a bowl.

2. Add the onion and garlic, and cook until starting to soften, about 5 minutes.

3. Return the sausage to the pot. Add the tomatoes, potatoes, beans, tomato sauce, broth, wine, basil, and oregano. Turn the heat to high and bring it to a boil, then turn to medium-low and simmer for 30 minutes.

4. Add the zucchini, tortellini and spinach and simmer 8 minutes more, or until the tortellini is cooked.

5. Serve the soup topped with grated Parmesan cheese.

Calories: 900 **Fat:** 44g **Carbs:** 72g **Fiber:** 10g **Sugar:** 13g **Protein:** 49g

---

Spicy Corn Chowder with Bacon

I added a can of pinto beans to give this tasty corn chowder more Mexican flair and an extra helping of filling fiber. Pureeing only half the soup concentrates the sweet corn flavor and adds creaminess while still leaving some satisfyingly chunky bites. To make it spicier, feel free to add more cayenne and/or leave the ribs and seeds in the jalapeños.

MAKES: 4 servings   **TOTAL TIME:** 45 minutes

6 slices bacon

1 white onion, chopped

1 red bell pepper, chopped

2 jalapeños, diced

1 teaspoon cayenne pepper

2 teaspoons salt

¼ cup all-purpose flour

2 Yukon gold potatoes, diced

1 (15-ounce) can pinto beans, drained

2 quarts chicken broth

16 ounces frozen corn or 1 (15-ounce) can whole kernel corn

1 cup heavy cream

1 avocado, peeled, pitted, and sliced

1. In a large stockpot or Dutch oven, cook the bacon over medium heat until crispy, about 5 to 6 minutes total. Remove to a paper towel–lined plate to cool, then roughly chop.

2. Add the onion, pepper, and jalapeños to the pot with the bacon fat. Cook until just starting to soften, about 5 minutes. Add the cayenne, salt, and flour, and cook, stirring, for 3 minutes.

3. Add the potatoes, beans, and chicken broth. Turn the heat to high and bring it to a boil, then turn to medium-low and simmer vigorously until the potatoes are tender, about 15 minutes.

4. Stir in the corn and cream, and simmer for 5 minutes, or until the frozen corn (if using) is heated through.

5. Transfer half the soup, or about 6 cups, to a blender and puree until mostly smooth. Return the pureed soup to the pot and stir to combine.

6. Serve the chowder topped with the chopped bacon and sliced avocado.

Calories: 770 **Fat:** 38g **Carbs:** 79g **Fiber:** 15g **Sugar:** 10g **Protein:** 35g

Mini Meatball Noodle Soup

I love the idea of scooping up a spoonful of soup and seeing one perfect, bite-size meatball swimming in the brothy goodness. Feel free to make these meatballs with any protein, such as ground turkey, chicken, pork, or lamb. I suggest browning them before cooking them through in the broth, but you can skip this step if you're short on time.

MAKES: 4 servings   **TOTAL TIME:** 50 minutes

1 pound ground beef

1 egg

½ cup breadcrumbs

1 cup grated Parmesan cheese, divided

2 teaspoons Italian seasoning, divided

2 teaspoons olive oil

6 carrots, peeled and chopped

4 celery stalks, chopped

2 quarts beef broth

1 teaspoon salt

2 tablespoons tomato paste

1 large zucchini, halved lengthwise and sliced

1 cup fresh or frozen peas

8 ounces whole wheat spaghetti, broken up into small pieces

2 cups fresh baby spinach

1. In a bowl, combine the ground beef, egg, breadcrumbs, ½ cup of grated Parmesan, and 1 teaspoon of Italian seasoning. Form the mixture into small meatballs, about 1½ inches in diameter.

2. In a large stockpot or Dutch oven, heat the olive oil over medium-high heat. Working in batches, brown the meatballs on all sides, about 4 minutes per batch. Set them aside as you brown them.

3. Add the carrots, celery, broth, salt, tomato paste, and remaining Italian seasoning to the pot. Turn the heat to high and bring it to a boil, scraping up any browned meatball bits, then turn to medium-low and simmer for 15 minutes.

4. Add the meatballs, zucchini, peas, and spaghetti. Turn the heat to medium and simmer until the spaghetti and meatballs are cooked, about 10 minutes.

5. Add the spinach and simmer for 5 minutes more.

6. Serve the soup topped with the remaining ½ cup of grated Parmesan.

Calories: 678 **Fat:** 18g **Carbs:** 65g **Fiber:** 11g **Sugar:** 13g **Protein:** 62g

Classic Chicken Noodle Soup

This is the Chicken Broth recipe from Chapter 5 (page 70) with a couple additions that make it the perfect soup for cold days, sick days, and any other days in between.

MAKES: 4 servings   **TOTAL TIME:** 2 hours 20 minutes

1 whole chicken, about 5 pounds, with skin, cut into pieces

4 quarts water

1 tablespoon kosher salt

4 carrots, peeled and chopped

2 parsnips, peeled and chopped

2 celery stalks, chopped

1 turnip, peeled and chopped

1 white onion, chopped

2 sprigs fresh dill

4 sprigs fresh parsley

1 (15-ounce) can cannellini beans, drained and rinsed

8 ounces whole wheat spaghetti, broken up into small pieces

1. Place the chicken pieces, water, and salt in a large stockpot. Cover and bring to a boil over high heat.

2. Add the carrots, parsnips, celery, turnip, and onion. Tie the dill and parsley together with cooking twine and add them to the pot. Cover, turn the heat to low, and simmer for 1½ hours. Add the beans and simmer for 30 minutes more.

3. Fish the chicken out of the pot. Pull the meat off the bones and return it to the soup. Add the spaghetti and simmer for 10 minutes, or until it is tender.

4. Remove the dill and parsley and serve.

Calories: 624 Fat: 12g **Carbs:** 74g **Fiber:** 15g **Sugar:** 11g **Protein:** 53g

Slow Cooker Beef Stew with Lentils

If you're going to spend a lazy Sunday at home, there's nothing better than simmering stew on the stove where you can constantly check in and smell it. But for days when that's not the case, the slow cooker is the perfect solution. This twist on a classic beef stew gets a fiber boost from chewy lentils.

MAKES: 6 servings   **TOTAL TIME:** 3 hours 40 minutes to 8 hours 40 minutes

2 tablespoons olive oil

2 pounds beef chuck roast or stew meat, cut into 1-inch chunks

6 carrots, peeled and sliced

2 Yukon gold potatoes, cut into chunks

1 large white onion, sliced

3 large cloves garlic, minced

4½ cups beef broth, divided

2 tablespoons tomato paste

1 tablespoon Worcestershire sauce

1 teaspoon dried rosemary

2 teaspoons dried thyme

1½ cups red lentils

¼ cup all-purpose flour

1. Heat the olive oil in a skillet over medium-high heat. Sear the beef in batches until it is browned on all sides, about 5 minutes per batch. Transfer the beef to the slow cooker.

2. Add the carrots, potatoes, onion, garlic, 4 cups of broth, tomato paste, Worcestershire sauce, rosemary, thyme, and lentils to the slow cooker and stir to combine. Cook on low for 6 to 8 hours or on high for 3 to 4 hours.

3. Thirty minutes before serving, whisk together the remaining ½ cup of broth and the flour and add it to the slow cooker. Turn

it to high (if it isn't there already) and cook for 30 minutes more.
Serve.

Calories: 899 Fat: 49g **Carbs:** 55g **Fiber:** 18g **Sugar:** 7g **Protein:** 59g

Slow Cooker Italian Chicken Stew

This is a spin on one of my favorite slow cooker recipes. The balsamic in the broth gives the stew an incredibly rich, delicious flavor.

MAKES: 4 servings   **TOTAL TIME:** 4 to 8 hours

K, GF

2 pounds boneless skinless chicken breast

salt, to taste

pepper, to taste

1 white onion, chopped

2 cups diced eggplant

4 cups chicken broth

½ cup balsamic vinegar

2 teaspoons Italian seasoning

1 teaspoon dried rosemary

1 teaspoon dried thyme

1 teaspoon dried oregano

3 large cloves garlic, minced

1 medium zucchini, halved lengthwise and sliced

10 ounces sliced mushrooms

1 (15-ounce) can cannellini beans, drained and rinsed

2 cups broccoli florets

1 cup grated Parmesan cheese, plus more for serving

1. Season the chicken with salt and pepper, and place it in a slow cooker. Add the onion, eggplant, broth, balsamic vinegar, Italian seasoning, rosemary, thyme, oregano, and garlic. Cook on low for 6 to 8 hours or on high for 4 to 6 hours.

2. Thirty minutes before serving, add the zucchini, mushrooms, cannellini beans, and broccoli. Turn it to high (if it isn't there already) and cook for 30 minutes more.

3. Remove the chicken, shred it, and return it to the slow cooker. Stir in the grated Parmesan cheese and serve with additional cheese for garnish.

Calories: 638 **Fat:** 22g **Carbs:** 24g **Fiber:** 9g **Sugar:** 7g **Protein:** 83g

Shrimp and Sausage Gumbo

The base of gumbo is called a roux, which is the combination of butter and flour that makes the stew thick and savory. You really do need to stir it constantly to keep it from burning, but trust me, it will be worth it!

MAKES: 4 servings   **TOTAL TIME:** 1 hour 15 minutes

1 pound andouille sausage, sliced

½ cup unsalted butter

½ cup all-purpose flour

1 white onion, diced

2 bell peppers, any color, diced

4 celery stalks, diced

3 large cloves garlic, minced

2 bay leaves

3 tablespoons Cajun seasoning blend

2 teaspoons cayenne pepper

2 quarts chicken broth

1 (14.5-ounce) can diced tomatoes

1 (15-ounce) can dark red kidney beans, drained and rinsed

2 cups long-grain brown rice

8 ounces fresh or frozen and thawed shrimp, peeled and deveined

2 green onions, sliced

1. In a large stockpot or Dutch oven over medium heat, cook the sausage until it is well browned, about 10 minutes. Remove to a bowl, leaving the fat in the pot.

2. Add the butter to the pot and stir until it is melted. Whisk in the flour, turn the heat to low and cook, whisking constantly, until it is a rich brown color, about 20 minutes.

3. Add the onion, bell peppers, celery, and garlic, and cook until soft, about 10 minutes.

4. Add the bay leaves, Cajun seasoning, cayenne, chicken broth, diced tomatoes, and kidney beans. Turn the heat to high and bring the mixture to a boil, then turn it to medium-low and simmer, partially covered and stirring occasionally, for at least 30 minutes.

5. Cook the rice according to the package instructions.

6. Stir in the shrimp with the gumbo ingredients and cook until they are opaque, about 5 minutes more.

7. Serve the gumbo over the rice and garnish with sliced green onions.

Calories: 1,294 **Fat:** 61g **Carbs:** 125g **Fiber:** 12g **Sugar:** 12g **Protein:** 64g

CHAPTER 11

Hearty Helpings

Chicken Pot Pie

This is my mom's chicken pot pie recipe that I've been enjoying my whole life. The only change I made was to use mixed frozen veggies instead of just peas and carrots to add some more variety. You can put this entire pie together through step 5 and then freeze it until you want to bake it. Serve it with a green salad for some extra freshness and crunch. This recipe is lower in fiber but makes up for it with a hefty serving of protein.

MAKES: 4 servings   **TOTAL TIME:** 1 hour 15 minutes

¾ pound boneless, skinless chicken breasts

1 (10-ounce) package mixed frozen veggies, like peas, carrots, and green beans

⅓ cup unsalted butter

⅓ cup all-purpose flour

¼ teaspoon onion powder

½ teaspoon salt, plus more to season chicken

¼ teaspoon pepper, plus more to season chicken

1¾ cups chicken broth

⅔ cup milk

2 refrigerated or frozen and thawed pie crusts

1. Preheat the oven to 350°F. Season the chicken with salt and pepper. Place it in an oven-safe dish and bake until cooked through, about 30 minutes. Remove and cut into bite-size pieces. Increase the oven temperature to 425°F.

2. Place the frozen veggies in a colander and rinse under cold water to separate.

3. In a medium saucepan, melt the butter over low heat. Stir in the flour, onion powder, ½ teaspoon of salt, and ¼ teaspoon of pepper and cook, stirring constantly, until bubbly, about 3 minutes.

4. Stir in the broth and milk. Bring to a boil, stirring often. Boil for 1 minute, then stir in the chicken and vegetables, and remove from the heat.

5. Grease a 9-inch pie plate. Lay one pie crust in the pie plate, pressing it into the bottom and up the sides. Pour in the filling and use a spatula to even out the top. Lay the second pie crust on top and pinch the edges together to seal.

6. Bake for 30 minutes or until the top crust is golden brown, and serve.

Calories: 1,106 **Fat:** 49g **Carbs:** 51g **Fiber:** 4g **Sugar:** 7g **Protein:** 106g

Pasta Bolognese with Easy Garlic Bread

The addition of mushrooms to this Bolognese sauce makes it extra thick, meaty, and filling. I like my Bolognese super thick, but if you like it thinner you can add some beef or chicken broth to get it to your desired consistency. The nutrition facts on this recipe include a few pieces of the garlic bread, which would also be delicious with the other pasta dishes in this chapter.

MAKES: 4 servings   **TOTAL TIME:** 1 hour 30 minutes

6 ounces cremini mushrooms

1 tablespoon olive oil

1 pound ground beef

1 large carrot, peeled and roughly chopped

½ medium yellow or sweet onion, roughly chopped

1 celery stalk, roughly chopped

2 cloves garlic, minced

2 teaspoons dried basil

2 teaspoons dried thyme

1 teaspoon salt

½ teaspoon pepper

½ cup red wine

1 (28-ounce) can crushed tomatoes

¼ cup heavy cream

1 pound whole wheat pasta, like rotini or tagliatelle

For the garlic bread:

1 French baguette

6 tablespoons unsalted butter, softened

4 large cloves garlic, crushed

1. Pulse the mushrooms about 10 times in a food processor to finely chop. Heat the olive oil in a large stockpot or Dutch oven over medium-high heat. Add the mushrooms and beef and cook, breaking up the meat with a wooden spoon, until the meat is no longer pink and the mushrooms have released their liquid, about 5 to 7 minutes. Use a slotted spoon to remove the beef and mushrooms from the pot and set aside, leaving any liquid in the pot.

2. Add the carrot, onion, and celery to a food processor and pulse 10 to 15 times to finely chop. Add them to the Dutch oven and cook over medium heat until they're soft, about 7 minutes.

3. Add the garlic, basil, thyme, salt, and pepper, and cook 1 minute. Add the wine and cook until most of the liquid is gone, about 3 minutes more.

4. Add the crushed tomatoes, cream, and beef and mushroom mixture to the pot. Bring to a simmer over medium, then turn the heat to low and simmer until the sauce has reduced and tightened, 1 hour.

5. When ready to eat, cook the pasta according to the package instructions. Top the pasta with some of the sauce. Serve with garlic bread.

For the garlic bread:

Preheat the oven to 250°F. Cut the baguette in half horizontally. Spread each half with 3 tablespoons of butter and 2 crushed cloves garlic. Place directly on the oven rack and toast just until the butter is melted and the bread begins to crisp up around the edges, about 8 minutes. Slice each half into 8 pieces and serve.

Calories: 1,325 **Fat:** 40g **Carbs:** 180g **Fiber:** 21g **Sugar:** 21g **Protein:** 57g

---

Skillet Pasta with Italian Sausage and Vodka Sauce

I am a huge fan of vodka sauce, marinara's lighter, sweeter, and creamier cousin. Chickpeas in pasta may seem a bit strange at first, but their mild flavor and slight chew blend perfectly into this quick and tasty dish.

MAKES: 4 servings   **TOTAL TIME:** 25 minutes

2 tablespoons olive oil, divided

1 pound sweet Italian sausage, casings removed

salt, to taste

pepper, to taste

1 medium head cauliflower, cut into florets

2 teaspoons Italian seasoning

1 pound whole wheat pasta, like penne or shells

1 (15-ounce) can chickpeas, drained and rinsed

1 (24-ounce) jar vodka sauce

2 ounces grated Parmesan cheese, plus more for serving

1. Heat 1 tablespoon of olive oil in a large, high-sided skillet over medium heat. Add the sausage, and season with salt and pepper. Cook, breaking up with a wooden spoon, until no longer pink, about 8 minutes. Remove from the pan and set aside.

2. Add the remaining tablespoon of olive oil to the skillet. Add the cauliflower florets and Italian seasoning, and cook until the cauliflower is cooked through and starting to brown on the edges, about 10 minutes.

3. Cook the pasta according to the package instructions. Drain.

4. Return the sausage to the skillet with the cauliflower. Add the chickpeas, pasta, vodka sauce, and Parmesan, and stir to combine. Turn the heat to medium-low and cook until everything is warmed through, about 2 minutes. Serve with more grated Parmesan.

Calories: 991 **Fat:** 31g **Carbs:** 132g **Fiber:** 18g **Sugar:** 19g **Protein:** 51g

Pesto Turkey Meatballs with Double Noodles

A few years ago, we started making meatballs with herby, garlicky pesto instead of eggs and never looked back. Adding zucchini noodles to whole wheat spaghetti increases the portion sizes for a satiety boost. Feel free to use ground beef instead of turkey if you'd prefer.

MAKES: 4 servings **TOTAL TIME:** 35 minutes

1 pound ground turkey

1 (5-ounce) container basil pesto

½ cup breadcrumbs

¼ cup milk

¼ cup grated Parmesan cheese, plus more for serving

1 pound whole wheat spaghetti

2 teaspoons olive oil

1 large or 2 small zucchini, thinly sliced or spiralized into noodles, or 2 cups prepared zucchini noodles

1 (24-ounce) jar marinara sauce

1. Preheat the oven to 400°F. In a bowl, mix together the ground turkey, pesto, breadcrumbs, milk, and Parmesan. Form 12 to 16 meatballs and place them on a large greased baking sheet. Bake for 20 to 22 minutes, until they are cooked through and crispy on the bottom. Turn off the oven but leave the meatballs inside to keep them warm.

2. Cook the whole wheat spaghetti in a large pot according to the package instructions. Drain and return to the pot.

3. Heat the olive oil in a skillet over medium. Use paper towels to squeeze as much moisture out of the zucchini noodles as you can. Add them to the skillet and sauté until they are just soft but not mushy, about 4 to 5 minutes.

4. Transfer the zucchini noodles to the pot with the hot spaghetti. Add the marinara sauce and toss to coat.

5. Place the noodles on a plate and top with some meatballs. Garnish with additional Parmesan and serve.

Calories: 848 **Fat:** 42g **Carbs:** 82g **Fiber:** 14g **Sugar:** 20g **Protein:** 56g

Chicken Marsala with Nutty Veggie Bowties

Chicken marsala is one of those dishes that I thought was complicated to make until the first time I tried my mom's recipe for it. Spoiler: it's actually a cinch! This recipe works best with thin chicken breasts, but you can also buy regular ones and pound them out. For a side, I wanted to create something reminiscent of rice pilaf but that would be more filling. Any shape pasta will work, but I like the way the bowties serve as an extra scoop for the veggies.

MAKES: 4 servings   **TOTAL TIME:** 40 minutes

1 pound boneless, skinless thin chicken breasts

flour, to coat chicken and thicken sauce

2 tablespoons olive oil, plus more for the veggies

1 pound cremini mushrooms, sliced

2 large cloves garlic, minced

1 tablespoon unsalted butter

¾ cup marsala wine

1 cup chicken broth

2 cups vegetable broth

1 pound whole wheat bow ties

½ sweet onion, diced

¾ cup fresh or frozen peas

2 carrots, peeled and diced

1 red bell pepper, cored and diced

¼ cup chopped walnuts

salt and pepper

1. Put the chicken and some flour in a large zip-top bag and toss to coat the chicken in the flour. Heat the olive oil in a large high-sided skillet over medium heat. Add the chicken and cook until lightly browned, about 4 minutes per side.

2. Move the chicken to the outside of the skillet. Add the mushrooms, garlic, and butter to the middle and cook until the mushrooms are soft, about 5 minutes.

3. Add the wine and broth to the skillet. Stir to mix everything together and cook until the sauce is thick, adding a teaspoon or two of flour as needed.

4. While the sauce is thickening, add the vegetable broth and 2 cups of water to a stockpot. Cook the bow ties according to the package instructions. Drain and set aside.

5. Add the onion, peas, carrots, bell pepper, and a splash of olive oil to the pot and cook until soft, about 8 minutes. Return the pasta to the pot, add the walnuts, and toss to combine. Season with salt and pepper.

6. Serve the chicken marsala alongside the pasta, all topped with the marsala sauce.

Calories: 918 **Fat:** 27g **Carbs:** 103g **Fiber:** 14g **Sugar:** 12g **Protein:** 58g

Kitchen Sink Enchiladas

Sure, there are the classic enchilada fillings, but you can truly wrap anything in a tortilla and smother it with sauce and cheese, and it will be delicious. This is one of my favorite combinations of fillings, but feel free to mix up the veggies or try pork butt or beef chuck roast in place of the chicken. Diced avocado or guacamole would also be delicious on top.

MAKES: 4 servings **TOTAL TIME:** 2½ to 5½ hours

GF

1 (15-ounce) can tomato sauce

1 tablespoon chipotle in adobo, minced

2 tablespoons chili powder

2 teaspoons ground cumin

3 large cloves garlic, minced

1 tablespoon dried minced onion

2 pounds boneless, skinless chicken breasts or thighs

salt, to taste

pepper, to taste

½ cup frozen corn

½ cup frozen peas

½ cup canned black beans, drained and rinsed

½ cup frozen broccoli florets, steamed according to package instructions

2 cups shredded jack cheese

12 (6-inch) corn tortillas

1. Combine the tomato sauce, chipotle in adobo, chili powder, cumin, garlic, and minced onion in the bowl of a slow cooker. Season the chicken with salt and pepper, and nestle it in the sauce. Cover and cook until the chicken is tender, 4 to 5 hours on low or 2 to 3 hours on high.

2. Remove the chicken to a cutting board and use two forks to shred it. Scoop ¾ cup of sauce out of the slow cooker and set it off to the side.

3. Return the chicken to the slow cooker. Add the corn, peas, black beans, broccoli, and half the cheese. Stir to combine and then place the cover back on to thaw the corn and peas.

4. Spray each tortilla on both sides with cooking spray. Stack them on a plate, cover them with a damp paper towel, and microwave them until soft, 1 minute.

5. Preheat the oven to 425°F. Coat the bottom of a 9 x 13-inch baking pan with some of the reserved sauce. Spoon filling into the center of a tortilla (I like to do this while holding the tortilla in my hand so the filling runs across my palm), roll it up, then place it in the pan seam-side down. Repeat with the remaining tortillas and filling.

6. Top the enchiladas with the remaining sauce and cheese. Grease a piece of aluminum foil with cooking spray and use it to cover the dish, greased side down. Bake 15 minutes or until the cheese is melted and serve.

Calories: 934 **Fat:** 27g **Carbs:** 90g **Fiber:** 16g **Sugar:** 13g **Protein:** 81g

Moroccan Tagine Chicken

This recipe is more of a chicken dish inspired by tagine than an actual tagine, which is more of a stew. Couscous and quinoa would also make great bases and you can use boneless chicken if you'd prefer. Don't forget to drizzle everything with the flavor-packed juice from the slow cooker before serving!

MAKES: 6 servings   **TOTAL TIME:** 4½ to 6½ hours

1 tablespoon olive oil

8 bone-in chicken thighs

salt, to taste

pepper, to taste

1 white onion, chopped

1 teaspoon ground cumin

¾ teaspoon ground coriander

¾ teaspoon ground cinnamon

½ teaspoon ground ginger

½ teaspoon ground turmeric

1 large clove garlic, minced

¼ cup raisins

¼ cup chopped dried apricots

3 carrots, peeled and chopped

1 (15-ounce) can chickpeas, drained and rinsed

1 cup chicken broth

2 cups brown rice

¼ cup slivered almonds

1. Heat the olive oil in a skillet over medium heat. Season the chicken with salt and pepper, and brown on both sides, about 3 minutes per side, then place it in a slow cooker. Add the onion to the pan and cook for 5 minutes to soften, then transfer to the slow cooker.

2. Add the spices, garlic, raisins, apricots, carrots, chickpeas, and chicken broth to the slow cooker and stir to mix. Cover and cook on low for 6 hours or high for 4 hours.

3. Cook the brown rice according to the package instructions.

4. Spread the slivered almonds on a small baking sheet or toaster oven tray. Heat the oven or toaster oven to 350°F. Add the almonds and toast (checking often, as these can burn very quickly) until the edges are just beginning to brown, about 3 minutes.

5. Serve the tagine over the rice and garnished with the toasted almonds, with some of the juice from the slow cooker drizzled over everything.

Calories: 912 **Fat:** 32g **Carbs:** 115g **Fiber:** 11g **Sugar:** 10g **Protein:** 41g

Beef, Spinach, and Pine Nut Un-Stuffed Shells

This casserole-esque recipe delivers all the goodness of stuffed shells with less work. If you use Parmesan cheese, make sure to use shredded, not grated, as it will melt into the sauce better and make it creamier.

MAKES: 6 servings   **TOTAL TIME:** 45 minutes

1 pound whole wheat pasta shells

2 teaspoons olive oil

1 pound ground beef

1 teaspoon Italian seasoning

salt, to taste

pepper, to taste

½ cup unsalted butter

1½ cups heavy cream

2 large cloves garlic, minced

½ teaspoon dried basil

½ teaspoon red pepper flakes

3 cups shredded Parmesan or Gruyere cheese, divided

5 ounces fresh baby spinach or 1 (8-ounce) package frozen spinach

½ cup pine nuts

1. Preheat the oven to 350°F. Cook the shells for 1 minute shorter than the package instructions. Drain well and transfer to a large bowl.

2. Heat the olive oil in a skillet over medium heat. Add the ground beef and Italian seasoning and season with salt and pepper. Cook, breaking up the meat with a wooden spoon, until browned and crumbly, about 8 minutes. Transfer to the bowl with the pasta.

3. Melt the butter in a medium saucepan over medium-low heat. Slowly whisk in the cream and simmer, whisking, about 3 minutes. Add the garlic, basil, and red pepper flakes and simmer for 1 minute. Add 2 cups of cheese and whisk constantly until melted and incorporated.

4. Pour the sauce into the bowl with the pasta and beef. Add the spinach and pine nuts and stir to mix everything together. Grease a 7 x 11-inch or 9 x 13-inch baking dish. Pour half the mixture in and top with ½ cup of the remaining cheese. Pour in the rest of the mixture and top with the remaining cheese. Bake for 25 minutes, until gooey and warmed through, and serve.

Calories: 1,063 **Fat:** 52g **Carbs:** 112g **Fiber:** 17g **Sugar:** 1g **Protein:** 50g

Barbecue Pulled Pork Sandwiches with Tangy Coleslaw

This pulled pork isn't overly sweet, nor is the coleslaw overly thick and heavy. I like lean pork tenderloin, but you could use a pork butt if you'd prefer. They mix in so well, you won't even notice the good-for-you flax seeds in the slaw!

MAKES: 4 servings   **TOTAL TIME:** 4 hours 10 minutes to 6 hours 10 minutes

2 pounds boneless pork tenderloin, cut into a few chunks

2 teaspoons plus ¼ cup olive oil, divided

1 cup ketchup

¼ cup molasses

4 teaspoons plus ¼ cup apple cider vinegar, divided

4 teaspoons Worcestershire sauce

2 teaspoons smoked paprika

½ teaspoon salt

¼ teaspoon pepper

1 tablespoon honey

1 teaspoon celery seed

1 (16-ounce) bag coleslaw mix

3 green onions, chopped

1 tablespoon flax seeds

4 whole wheat hamburger buns

1. In a skillet over medium-high heat, heat 2 teaspoons of olive oil. Sear the pork until it is browned on all sides, then transfer to a slow cooker.

2. Add the ketchup, molasses, 4 teaspoons of apple cider vinegar, Worcestershire sauce, smoked paprika, salt, and pepper to the slow cooker. Stir to combine and coat the pork. Cook on low for 6 hours or high for 4 hours.

3. In a large bowl, whisk the remaining olive oil and apple cider vinegar with the honey and celery seed. Add the coleslaw mix, green onions, and flax seeds, and toss to coat. Cover and chill in the fridge until ready to serve.

4. Remove the pork from the slow cooker and use two forks to shred it. Give the sauce a quick stir, then return the pork to the slow cooker and toss it with the sauce.

5. Toast your buns, if you'd like, then top with pulled pork. Serve with the coleslaw on top of the pork or alongside.

Calories: 1,044 **Fat:** 32g **Carbs:** 74g **Fiber:** 9g **Sugar:** 46g **Protein:** 113g

Garlicky Pasta with Eggplant, Artichokes, and Mushrooms

Canned artichoke hearts are much easier to work with than whole artichokes, but make sure you buy plain ones and not marinated, which can add an unpleasant acidity to this dish. This is one recipe that will benefit from using fresh garlic as opposed to dried or jarred. If you're a big fan of garlic (like I am), feel free to add two or three more cloves for more of the savory delicious flavor.

MAKES: 4 servings   **TOTAL TIME:** 20 minutes

1 pound whole wheat pasta, like rotini

1 medium eggplant, cut into 1-inch pieces

¼ cup olive oil

4 large cloves garlic, chopped

2 teaspoons Italian seasoning

1 cup canned artichoke hearts, chopped

12 ounces sliced mushrooms

1 small zucchini, cut into 1-inch pieces

1 cup vegetable broth

1 cup Parmesan cheese

¼ cup chopped walnuts

1. Cook the pasta according to the package instructions. Drain and keep warm.

2. Place the eggplant in a single layer on a paper towel–lined plate. Microwave on high for 3 minutes.

3. Meanwhile, heat the olive oil in a large high-sided skillet over medium-low heat. Add the garlic and Italian seasoning, and cook until the garlic softens and browns, about 6 minutes.

4. Add the eggplant, artichokes, mushrooms, zucchini, and vegetable broth to the skillet. Turn the heat to medium and cook for 3 minutes. Stir in the Parmesan cheese and pasta, cover, and cook for 2 minutes more.

5. Serve the pasta garnished with the chopped walnuts and more Parmesan, if desired.

Calories: 732 **Fat:** 25g **Carbs:** 107g **Fiber:** 20g **Sugar:** 14g **Protein:** 26g

Spinach and Zucchini Lasagna

You can make lasagna with regular noodles and you can make it with zucchini noodles. Why not make it with both? Make sure you don't cut the zucchini too thin or it will shrink up to nothing when you roast it.

MAKES: 4 servings   **TOTAL TIME:** 1 hour 30 minutes

2 medium zucchini

2 teaspoons olive oil, plus more for drizzling

1 pound ground beef

1 teaspoon dried basil

1 (15-ounce) container ricotta cheese

1 cup grated Parmesan cheese

1 large egg

1 cup fresh basil leaves, shredded

9 oven-ready lasagna noodles, whole wheat if possible

1 (8-ounce) package frozen spinach, thawed, drained, and water squeezed out

1 (28-ounce) jar marinara sauce

2 cups shredded mozzarella cheese

salt and pepper

1. Preheat the oven to 425°F. Slice the zucchini length-wise into ½-inch-thick strips. Spread on a baking sheet, sprinkle with salt, and let it sit at least 10 minutes or up to 30 minutes.

2. Pour off any water and pat the zucchini dry with paper towels. Drizzle with a little olive oil or spray it with olive oil spray and roast for 25 minutes. Remove and turn the oven down to 350°F.

3. While the zucchini is roasting, heat the 2 teaspoons of olive oil in a skillet over medium heat. Add the ground beef, dried basil, and a pinch of salt and pepper and cook, breaking up the beef into crumbles, until it is cooked through, about 8 minutes.

4. In a bowl, combine the ricotta, Parmesan, egg, and fresh basil.

5. Spread some marinara sauce in the bottom of a 13 x 9-inch baking dish. Lay down three lasagna noodles, followed by a layer of zucchini, then beef, then spinach, then sauce, then ricotta mixture, then shredded cheese. Repeat two more times.

6. Cover the pan with aluminum foil and bake for 30 minutes. Remove the foil and bake for 10 minutes more. Remove the lasagna and let it sit for at least 10 minutes before serving.

Calories: 784 **Fat:** 30g **Carbs:** 71g **Fiber:** 13g **Sugar:** 21g **Protein:** 59g

Sweet Potato Shepherd's Pie with Lentils

This shepherd's pie is incredibly hearty, thanks to the fiber-rich lentils hidden in the filling. To make spreading the sweet potatoes easier, spray a spatula with cooking spray and use it to spread the potatoes over the filling.

MAKES: 4 servings   **TOTAL TIME:** 45 minutes

GF

½ cup black or red lentils

4 large sweet potatoes

1 tablespoon olive oil

1 pound ground beef

1 sweet onion, chopped

4 carrots, peeled and chopped

5 ounces sliced mushrooms

4 tablespoons tomato paste

½ teaspoon ground nutmeg

2 teaspoons chili powder

2 tablespoons unsalted butter

1. Preheat the oven to 375°F. Cook the lentils according to the package instructions. Drain well.

2. While the lentils are cooking, pierce the potatoes a few times with a fork. Place them on a microwave-safe plate and microwave for 10 to 12 minutes, until tender.

3. Heat the oil in a medium oven-safe skillet over medium heat. Add the ground beef, onion, carrots, and mushrooms, and cook, breaking up the beef with a wooden spoon, until everything is cooked and soft, about 10 minutes. Drain about 1 tablespoon of liquid from the pan, but not all.

4. Stir in the tomato paste, nutmeg, chili powder, and lentils, and turn the heat to low.

5. When the potatoes are cool enough to handle, scoop out the insides and mash them with the butter until smooth (you can also use a food processor for this step).

6. Spread the potato mixture on top of the meat mixture. Bake for 20 minutes, until heated through. Serve.

Calories: 660 **Fat:** 17g **Carbs:** 80g **Fiber:** 19g **Sugar:** 8g **Protein:** 46g

---

Mexican-Style Pulled Pork Tacos with Spicy Guacamole

Inspired by an *America's Test Kitchen* recipe, this sweet and spicy sauce is a play on *mole*, but faster and with fewer ingredients. If you don't have time or don't want to make your own guacamole, feel free to pick up some that's already made.

MAKES: 4 servings   **TOTAL TIME:** 6 hours 10 minutes to 8 hours 10 minutes

GF

1 (15-ounce) can tomato sauce

1 cup raisins

2 tablespoons chili powder

1 tablespoon ground cumin

1 tablespoon creamy peanut butter

1 tablespoon unsweetened cocoa powder

3 large cloves garlic

2 pounds pork butt roast, cut into a few pieces

salt, to taste

pepper, to taste

2 avocados

¼ cup minced fresh cilantro

1 teaspoon minced chipotle in adobo

1 lime

8 corn tortillas

¼ red onion, thinly sliced

½ cup white or red cabbage

1. In a slow cooker, combine the tomato sauce, raisins, chili powder, cumin, peanut butter, cocoa powder, and garlic. Season the pork with salt and pepper, nestle in the sauce, and cook for 8 to 10 hours on low or 6 to 7 hours on high.

2. Remove the pork to a bowl and shred it. Using an immersion blender or regular blender, process the sauce until it is smooth. Toss the pork with the sauce.

3. In a bowl, mash together the avocadoes, cilantro, chipotle in adobo, the juice of half a lime, and salt to taste.

4. Brush or spray the tortillas on both sides with olive oil and stack them on a plate. Drape a damp paper towel over them and microwave for 40 seconds to soften.

5. Scoop some of the pork onto each tortilla. Top with the guacamole, sliced onion, and cabbage, and drizzle with lime juice to serve.

Calories: 948 **Fat:** 40g **Carbs:** 74g **Fiber:** 16g **Sugar:** 29g **Protein:** 81g

Recipe Index

Conversions

Volume

U.S.	U.S. Equivalent	Metric
1 tablespoon (3 teaspoons)	½ fluid ounce	15 milliliters
¼ cup	2 fluid ounces	60 milliliters
⅓ cup	3 fluid ounces	90 milliliters
½ cup	4 fluid ounces	120 milliliters
⅔ cup	5 fluid ounces	150 milliliters
¾ cup	6 fluid ounces	180 milliliters
1 cup	8 fluid ounces	240 milliliters
2 cups	16 fluid ounces	480 milliliters

Weight

U.S.	Metric
½ ounce	15 grams
1 ounce	30 grams
2 ounces	60 grams
¼ pound	115 grams
⅓ pound	150 grams
½ pound	225 grams
¾ pound	350 grams
1 pound	450 grams

Temperature

Fahrenheit (°F)	Celsius (°C)
70°F	20°C
100°F	40°C
120°F	50°C
130°F	55°C
140°F	60°C
150°F	65°C
160°F	70°C
170°F	75°C
180°F	80°C
190°F	90°C
200°F	95°C
220°F	105°C
240°F	115°C
260°F	125°C
280°F	140°C
300°F	150°C
325°F	165°C
350°F	175°C
375°F	190°C
400°F	200°C
425°F	220°C
450°F	230°C

Acknowledgments

First, I need to thank Ulysses Press for giving me the opportunity to write my first book. To Casie Vogel, thank you for your patience and for believing in me for this project. To Bridget Thoreson, thank you for your feedback and support as I was writing. Writing a book is a huge undertaking, and you both gave me the confidence and encouragement to do it.

To Melissa Sorrells, my work-wife turned forever-friend, thank you for always being there when I needed to float an idea or discuss a study. Knowing you are just a Gchat away is a constant source of comfort. To Jennifer Joseph, thank you for teaching me how to write clearly and knowledgably about nutrition and food. Without your tutelage, I would never have had the wherewithal or the confidence to take on this project in the first place. And to Carol Brooks, thank you for giving me my first opportunity to do this work of helping and educating people through words. I will be forever grateful.

To my family: Mom, Dad, Jess, Jake, Nan, Grandma, Grandpa, and everyone else up in New England, thank you for always believing in me, and for your excitement for me as I took on this project. Knowing that you are always in my corner, even though you're a few states away, keeps me going every day.

Finally, to my husband, Jeff—your support, positivity, and love hold me up. Thank you for trying my recipes when I needed to test them, for entertaining Copper when I needed to focus, and for always cheering me on. I couldn't do any of what I do without you.

About the Author

Alyssa Sybertz is a freelance journalist and copywriter with an expertise in health, nutrition, fitness, and food. She is a regular contributor to *Woman's World* and *FIRST for Women*, the top two retail magazines in the US, and is the food editor at *Closer Weekly*. She has written for Allrecipes.com, *WholeFoods Magazine,* and various global wellness brands, plus authored comprehensive guides on health-related topics for nationwide marketing campaigns. Alyssa is a certified Zumba instructor and enjoys hiking, snowboarding, and trying new recipes. She lives outside of Washington, D.C., with her husband and her dog, Copper. You can find her at AlyssaSybertz. com. This is her first book.